*Mickey C. Smith*
*Editor*

# Pharmaceutical Marketing in the 21st Century

*Pre-publication*
*REVIEWS,*
*COMMENTARIES,*
*EVALUATIONS . . .*

"**I**n every field there is a leader. Once in a great while, that leader is able to assemble in one place the state-of-the-art information about her/his field. Mickey Smith has done just this in *Pharmaceutical Marketing in the 21st Century.*

The text is easy to read, informative and, most important, applicable to almost any size pharma business.

I would especially like to call the reader's attention to Steve Chappell's introduction, since there are few individuals in our industry who have the perspective and the facts to present as well as Steve does.

This has to be required reading for everyone who works in healthcare."

**Ted Klein, B.S./M.A.**
*President, Ted Klein & Company*
*Chairman, MMD, Inc.*

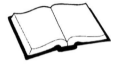

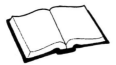

Pharmaceutical Products Press
An Imprint of
The Haworth Press, Inc.
New York • London

# Pharmaceutical Marketing in the 21st Century

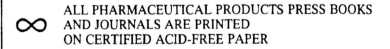

# Pharmaceutical Marketing in the 21st Century

Mickey C. Smith
Editor

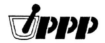

Pharmaceutical Products Press
An Imprint of
The Haworth Press, Inc.
New York • London

Published by

Pharmaceutical Products Press, 10 Alice Street, Binghamton, NY 13904-1580 USA

Pharmaceutical Products Press, an imprint of The Haworth Press, Inc., 10 Alice Street, Binghamton, NY 13904-1580 USA

*Pharmaceutical Marketing in the 21st Century* has also been published as *Journal of Pharmaceutical Marketing & Management*, Volume 10, Numbers 2/3/4 1996.

The development, preparation, and publication of this work has been undertaken with great care. However, the publisher, employees, editors, and agents of The Haworth Press and all imprints of The Haworth Press, Inc., including The Haworth Medical Press and Pharmaceutical Products Press, are not responsible for any errors contained herein or for consequences that may ensue from use of materials or information contained in this work. Opinions expressed by the author(s) are not necessarily those of The Haworth Press, Inc.

Paperback edition published in 1997.

Cover design by Stephanie Torta.

**Library of Congress Cataloging-in-Publication Data**

Pharmaceutical marketing in the 21st century / Mickey Smith, editor
    p.   cm.
    "Has also been published as Journal of pharmaceutical marketing & management, volume 10, numbers 2/3/4, 1996"–T.p. verso.
    Includes bibliographical references.
    ISBN 0-7890-0207-8 (alk. paper)
    1. Drugs–Marketing.  I. Smith, Mickey C.
    [DNLM: 1. Drug Industry–economics.  2. Marketing of Health Services–trends.  3. Pharmacy Administration.  W1 J0892H v. 10 no. 2/3 1996 / QV 736 P53605 1996]
HD9665.5.P524  1996
615.1'068'8–dc20
DNLM/DLC
for Library of Congress                                                                       95-26641
                                                                                                          CIP

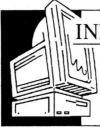

# INDEXING & ABSTRACTING

Contributions to this publication are selectively indexed or abstracted in print, electronic, online, or CD-ROM version(s) of the reference tools and information services listed below. This list is current as of the copyright date of this publication. See the end of this section for additional notes.

- *ABI/INFORM Global (broad-coverage indexing & abstracting service that includes numerous English- language titles outside the USA available from University Microfilms International (UMI), 300 North Zeeb Road, PO Box 1346, Ann Arbor, MI 48106-1346)*, UMI Data Courier, Attn: Library Services, Box 34660, Louisville, KY 40232

- *ABSCAN, Inc.,* P.O. Box 2384, Monroe, LA 71207-2384

- *Biosciences Information Service of Biological Abstracts (BIOSIS),* Biosciences Information Service, 2100 Arch Street, Philadelphia, PA 19103-1399

- *Cabell's Directory of Publishing Opportunities in Business & Economics (comprehensive & descriptive bibliographic listing with editorial criteria and publication production data for selected business & economics journals),* Cabell Publishing Company, Box 5428, Tobe Hahn Station, Beaumont, TX 77726-5428

- *CNPIEC Reference Guide: Chinese National Directory of Foreign Periodicals,* P.O. Box 88, Beijing, Peoples Republic of China

- *Human Resources Abstracts HRA,* Sage Publications, Inc., 2455 Teller Road, Newbury Park, CA 91320

(continued)

- *InPharma Weekly DIGEST & NEWS on: Pharmaceutical Literature, Drug Reactions & LMS*, Adis International Ltd., 41 Centorian Drive, Mairangi Bay, Auckland 10, New Zealand

- *International Pharmaceutical Abstracts,* American Society of Hospital Pharmacists, 7272 Wisconsin Avenue, Bethesda, MD 20814

- *INTERNET ACCESS (& additional networks) Bulletin Board for Libraries ("BUBL"), coverage of information resources on INTERNET, JANET, and other networks.*
  - JANET X.29: UK.AC.BATH.BUBL or 80006012101300
  - TELNET: BUBL.BATH.AC.UK or 138.38.32.45 login 'bubl'
  - Gopher: BUBL.BATH.AC.UK (138.32.32.45). Port 7070
  - World Wide Web: http: / / www.bubl.bath.ac.uk./BUBL/ home.html
  - NISSWAIS telnetniss.ac. uk (for the NISS gateway),
  The Andersonian Library, Curran Building, 101 St. James Road, Glasgow G4 ONS, Scotland

- *Management & Marketing Abstracts,* Pira International, Randalls Road, Leatherhead, Surrey KT22 7RU, England

- *Medical Benefits,* P.O. Box 1007, Charlottesville, VA 22902

- *Medication Use STudies (MUST) DATABASE,* The University of Mississippi, School of Pharmacy, University, MS 38677

- *Pharmacy Business,* Southeastern University, 1750 NE 168th Street, North Miami Beach, FL 33162

- *Public Affairs Information Bulletin (PAIS),* Public Affairs Information Service, Inc., 521 West 43rd Street, New York, NY 10036-4396

(continued)

# SPECIAL BIBLIOGRAPHIC NOTES

*related to special journal (separates)*
*and indexing/abstracting*

- [ ] indexing/abstracting services in this list will also cover material in any "separate" that is co-published simultaneously with Haworth's special thematic journal issue or DocuSerial. Indexing/abstracting usually covers material at the article/chapter level.

- [ ] monographic co-editions are intended for either nonsubscribers or libraries which intend to purchase a second copy for their circulating collections.

- [ ] monographic co-editions are reported to all jobbers/wholesalers/approval plans. The source journal is listed as the "series" to assist the prevention of duplicate purchasing in the same manner utilized for books-in-series.

- [ ] to facilitate user/access services all indexing/abstracting services are encouraged to utilize the co-indexing entry note indicated at the bottom of the first page of each article/chapter/contribution.

- [ ] this is intended to assist a library user of any reference tool (whether print, electronic, online, or CD-ROM) to locate the monographic version if the library has purchased this version but not a subscription to the source journal.

- [ ] individual articles/chapters in any Haworth publication are also available through the Haworth Document Delivery Services (HDDS).

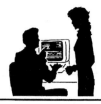

# ABOUT THE EDITOR

**Mickey C. Smith, Ph.D.,** F.A.P. Barnard Distinguished Professor, is Associate Director of the Bureau of Pharmaceutical Services, Research Professor in the Research Institute of Pharmaceutical Sciences, and Professsor of Management and Marketing in the School of Businesss at the University of Mississippi, and an adjunct faculty member of the University of Tennessee School of Pharmacy and the University of Alabama School of Public Health. A highly acclaimed researcher/writer with an international reputation in the pharmaceutical marketing field, Dr. Smith has published more than 350 research and professional articles in more than 100 journals and is the author of 8 books, 4 of which are in multiple editions and 1 of which has been translated and published in Japan and Spain. He serves as editor of the *Journal of Pharmaceutical Marketing & Management* and the *Journal of Research in Pharmaceutical Economics*, and is on the editorial boards of other national and international journals.

# Pharmaceutical Marketing in the 21st Century

## CONTENTS

# EDITOR'S NOTE

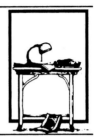

Some of those reading this material will have received it as part of a subscription to the *Journal of Pharmaceutical Marketing & Management*. Others will be reading from a book, *Pharmaceutical Marketing in the 21st Century*. Regardless of the circumstances, this collection of papers is, we believe, extraordinary. A distinguished group of contributors has provided a fascinating and diverse set of opinions about what may lie ahead for this exciting industry.

Given the rate of change in the pharmaceutical industry today, it takes near temerity to predict anything more than two weeks in the future. But we believe the reader will agree that the contributors have used a combination of history, experience, and imagination to provide an interesting glimpse into the possible future.

This publication marks the end of ten years of *JPMM*. We are pleased to have been a part of this and extend the most sincere appreciation to the editorial board members, authors, reviewers, and subscribers. The staff of Haworth Press, and especially the publisher, as well as the managing editor, Julie Fisher, have made this a very rewarding experience for the editor and, we trust, the reader.

*Mickey Smith*
*Editor*

[Haworth co-indexing entry note]: "Editor's Note." Smith, Mickey C. Co-published simultaneously in *Journal of Pharmaceutical Marketing & Management* (Pharmaceutical Products Press, an imprint of The Haworth Press, Inc.) Vol. 10, No. 2/3, 1996, p 1; and *Pharmaceutical Marketing in the 21st Century* (ed: Mickey C. Smith): Pharmaceutical Products Press, an imprint of The Haworth Press, Inc., 1996, p. 1. Single or multiple copies of this article are available from The Haworth Document Delivery Service [1-800-342-9678, 9:00 a.m. - 5:00 p.m. (EST)].

# INVITED PAPERS

# Global Pharma 20/20

William R. Mattson, Jr.
Evan G. Dick

## *LOOKING BACK 20 YEARS*

*The best of prophets of the future is the past.* – Lord Byron, 1821.

It's 1975, and the World Pharmaceutical Market approaches $30 billion. Antibiotics are the leading therapeutic category at $5+ billion; cardiovasculars are under $4 billion. The U.S. market is the largest in the world at $6.5 billion; Japan ($3.3 billion), Germany ($3 billion), and France ($2.5 billion) are next. The hot growth prospects are Japan, Latin America, and the Middle East.

As we look back 20 years, the leading companies (all with 1-2% shares) are Roche, Merck, Sandoz, Lilly, and Wyeth. Glaxo did not appear in the top ten due mainly to its absence from the U.S. market. Driving company

---

William R. Mattson, Jr., is President of The Mattson Jack Group, 11960 Westline Industrial Drive, St. Louis, MO 63146. Evan G. Dick, Ph.D., is Vice President and General Manager at MedStrategy Management Reports, 11960 Westline Industrial Drive, St. Louis, MO 63146.

[Haworth co-indexing entry note]: "Global Pharma 20/20." Mattson, William R., and Evan G. Dick. Co-published simultaneously in *Journal of Pharmaceutical Marketing & Management* (Pharmaceutical Products Press, an imprint of The Haworth Press, Inc.) Vol. 10, No. 2/3, 1996, pp. 3-18; and *Pharmaceutical Marketing in the 21st Century* (ed: Mickey C. Smith) Pharmaceutical Products Press, an imprint of The Haworth Press, Inc., 1996, pp. 3-18. Single or multiple copies of this article are available from The Haworth Document Delivery Service [1-800-342-9678, 9:00 a.m. - 5:00 p.m. (EST)].

*3*

performance are the top products: Valium® (a $300+ million product), Hydergine®, Aldomet®, Keflex®, and many other cephalosporin brands.

## TODAY'S BASELINE

Fast forward 20 years to 1995. The world market is eight- to ninefold higher–$250 billion and expected to hit $350 billion by 2000. Cardiovasculars alone total nearly $30 billion, equal to the total market in 1975 and nearly twice the size of the global antibiotic market. New therapeutic categories driving overall market growth such as quinolones, ACE inhibitors, calcium channel blockers, and HMG-CoA reductase inhibitors did not exist in 1975. Combined, these categories alone exceed the total market in 1975. These are some of the products of the pharmaceutical industry innovation, which required decades of creativity, development, and funding.

The U.S. market continues to be the largest at $70 billion (1993), fueled by the double-digit growth of the 1980s, primarily through price increases. Japan, the reunited Germany, France, and Italy are next; this is the same rank order as 20 years ago. The hot growth markets recently are the Tiger States of Korea, Indonesia, Thailand, India et al., and China. North America is the same size as "united" Europe. Latin America has fallen in importance. Soon the Tiger States will surpass it (Figure 1).

The leading pharmaceutical companies in 1995 are Glaxo, with its recent purchase of Wellcome; Hoechst, with its pending purchase of Marion Merrell Dow; Merck, Bristol-Myers Squibb, SmithKline Beecham, and

FIGURE 1. World Market Share by Region, 1993.

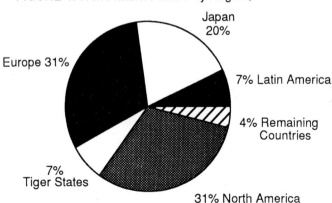

Source: Definitive Data Tactics, UK, 1994 Global Pharma Market Review

Johnson & Johnson. Roche, Wyeth, Sandoz, and Lilly have dropped in ranking despite their several acquisitions. Concentration is ongoing; however, the leading companies have 3-5% market shares, and the industry is still not a heavily concentrated one by any standard. Other changes are that 4 Japanese companies rank in the Top 30, but still mainly with sales from the home market. These companies haven't yet penetrated foreign markets, despite the push by their government to do so.

Nearly 20 pharmaceutical brands exceeded (or will soon exceed) $1 billion by 1993, with Zantac approaching $4 billion (Table 1). All of these global brands debuted since 1975; however, a few of the Top 25 were important brands then and are still today (Premarin®, Tylenol®, and Ventolin®).

These brands and some other product life extension miracles (e.g., Abbott's macrolide franchise) make one pause to contemplate the wisdom of long-range investment in expansion of indications, proliferation of line extensions, company franchise and image development, conversions from prescription to over-the-counter (Rx to OTC), and globalization of brands. How many of these Top 50 products will still appear as leading brands in 20 years? What can be done to prolong their life cycles?

## *LOOKING FORWARD 20 YEARS*

Fast forward 20 years to 2015, with 20/20 vision. The fact that no one knows anything about the future makes all business forecasters much more sure.

Many therapeutic classes have disappeared as a result of gene therapy for several diseases. We have new rational therapies for the prevention and treatment of myocardial infarction, stroke, and AIDS (which has been controlled, at least in the developed world).

The leading countries in the global market are the U.S., Japan, China (new entrant), Germany, Italy, and France. The leading companies? Who knows? Too many mega merger companies have blurred this vision. The survivors are those with strong pharmaceutical R&D and health care balance (not just dependent on pharmaceuticals). Still, the largest company will have less than a 10% market share.

The leading products are probably those treating the remaining unserved/underserved conditions of today: stroke, AIDS, M.I., obesity, and asthma, among others. Especially important will be those medications that treat geriatric conditions, extending and improving life after 65 for the baby-boomer generation.

TABLE 1. Twenty-five Leading Global Products, 1989-1993.

| $U.S. (mil.) | 1989 | 1993 |
|---|---|---|
| Zantac | 2,538 | 3,804 |
| Vasotec/ Renitec | 1,183 | 1,922 |
| Zovirax | 596 | 1,380 |
| Voltaren | 1,049 | 1,300 |
| Prozac | 407 | 1,235 |
| Augmentin | 553 | 1,230 |
| Procardia | 486 | 1,197 |
| Capoten | 1,001 | 1,166 |
| Ciproxin | 475 | 1,166 |
| Ceclor | 797 | 1,121 |
| Tagamet | 1,159 | 1,109 |
| Cardizem | 838 | 1,107 |
| Mevacor | 530 | 1,107 |
| Adalat | 965 | 1,100 |
| Losec | 31 | 940 |
| Mevalotin | 36 | 939 |
| Zocor | 69 | 928 |
| Naprosyn | 765 | 892 |
| Rocephin | 490 | 805 |
| Ventolin | 577 | 790 |
| Becotide | 425 | 766 |
| Premarin | 316 | 747 |
| Pepcid/Pepcidine | 377 | 715 |
| Tylenol | 620 | 700 |
| Sandimmune | 369 | 680 |

Source: Definitive Data Tactics, UK, 1994 Gobal Pharma Market Review

## WATERSHED EVENTS/TRENDS SINCE 1975

*He that will not apply new remedies must expect new evils; for time is the greatest innovator.* – Francis Bacon, 1625

What, then, are those events/trends of the last 20 years that defined where we are today and that will continue to affect our business over the next 20 years? Table 2 summarizes them. Let's look at some of those that will continue to affect the industry's course over the next 20 years.

One mentor gave me some sage advice during my early career at Abbott International: "Be kind and respectful to all, even your competitor, because you never know whether you'll be working for them." Truer words could not have been spoken given the mega merger trends in the last ten years. The census of substantial companies has been reduced by approximately 50%. Remember Richardson-Merrell, Robins, Erbamont, Syntex, Lederle, and Sterling-Winthrop? All of these and many more were integrated into successor companies, some several times!

We also learned how to collaborate with our competition, which will certainly continue to be the rule and not the exception during the next 20 years. The single most successful licensing deal ever made in the global pharmaceutical industry is the Glaxo-Roche Zantac® copromotion deal. It catapulted Glaxo from nowhere to #2 in the U.S. in one decade, Roche from the edge of the abyss caused by the Valium patent expiration to

TABLE 2. Twenty Watershed Events/Trends Since 1975.

| Commercial | Scientific/Technical |
|---|---|
| • Mega mergers | • Recombinant DNA/RNA technologies |
| • Zantac co-promotion | • Gene identification/modification-therapeutics |
| • Japan Inc. globalization | • Receptor-driven drug discovery |
| • Price controls–Europe/Japan | • Monoclonal antibodies–diagnostics |
| • Flag planting/retreating | • Rational drug design methodologies |
| • Rise and fall of pharma industry profits and valuations | • Breakthrough research in immunology and neuroscience |
| • Emergence of biotech industry | • Innovative drug delivery systems |
| • Rise of generics–U.S. et al. | • Escalation of R&D cost and time |
| • Puerto Rico/Ireland tax shelters | • "Harmonization" of clinical research to co-serve U.S. and European regulatory needs |
| • Managed care power | • Combinatorial chemistry |

global prosperity, and SmithKline into the arms of Beecham, a transatlantic merger that enabled the two companies to avoid being acquired by others.

### NEW DIRECTIONS–AWAY FROM HOME

No other industry is as global as pharmaceuticals. Figure 2 portrays what we have seen over the last two decades. European companies invading the U.S., Japanese companies going off-shore in both directions, and U.S. companies selectively going overseas. What's missing? The remaining developed markets (Canada, Australia, South Africa et al.), the chronically troubled markets (Latin America, the previous Soviet Block, and the Middle East), and the developing world (Africa, China, India, and selected Asian markets such as Indonesia, Thailand et al.).

In the 1970s, we raced to plant flags everywhere. Remember the great market opportunities of Iran, Saudi Arabia, and Brazil where "its greatness will forever be 20 years ahead?" In the 1980s, U.S. multinationals retreated. Many multinationals announced with pride that they were focusing on only 8-10 countries, having sold/licensed their business elsewhere. European and selected Japanese companies, especially those with strong chemical/agricultural legs, stayed and now stand to prosper. Perhaps so, but in our lifetimes? Patience and vision are often rewarded, but not always.

### THE 1980s–GOLDEN YEARS?

This strategy of geographic concentration, especially in the U.S. with its "free pricing," led to the unprecedented rise in the profitability and

FIGURE 2. Globalization of the Pharmaceutical Industry.

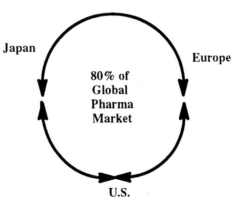

valuation of the global pharmaceutical industry. How many pharmaceutical companies appeared on the 1992 list of the 100 most valuable industrial companies in the world as measured in market capitalization? Over 20! This was, of course, after a decade of double-digit U.S. price increases and before the power of managed care and the election of the Clintons.

Pricing in the U.S.–the ultimate lever of global profitability during the 1980s, when teamed with Puerto Rican and other tax shelter benefits–led to an industry arms race and a public relations black eye. Without this pricing component of growth, our many other strategies would not have the fuel to proceed. Little did our ultimate customer, the patient, and other constituencies (managed care and Washington) remember that we didn't raise prices at all in the 1970s or that our R&D expense is galloping up due to new regulatory requirements for larger and longer studies. Admittedly, we sure didn't explain ourselves very well to John Q. Public. If only the industry had invested in global public relations to explain its benefits and not just describe its features, such as high R&D.

Our troops in the trenches, our sales representative forces, multiplied 2 or 3 times for most companies over the last 20 years, primarily in the U.S. We concentrated on reach and frequency, à la consumer products. We even borrowed other companies' representative forces to launch new products. It became the rule, not the exception, to copromote in the U.S., Japan, and selected European countries. Now we find ourselves in the position of ratcheting down these rep forces or consolidating them as the power of the individual physician is constrained under managed care.

## SCIENTIFIC PROGRESS SINCE 1975–
## HIGH RISKS & HIGH REWARDS

Twenty years ago, the pharmaceutical industry joined academe, agriculture, and other industries at the threshold of an anticipated era of molecular biology, of having ready access to nature's most closely held secrets. The step over the threshold took place, and with revolutionary power, advances in both DNA and protein chemistry have fundamentally reshaped the drug discovery landscape. The pace of new discoveries is already challenging the capacity of our industry to absorb them, and this pace will quicken with the advent of new methodologies such as combinatorial chemistry.

The advances of the past two decades can be unashamedly described as a testimony to the human spirit, dogged hard work, broad government support of basic research, and aggressive commercial risk investment in cutting-edge science. While drug discovery efforts in many fields (e.g., neuroscience, endocrinology, immunology) have been carried forward on a worldwide tide of advancing technical methods, molecular biology has acted as a discovery booster rocket for both diagnostics and drugs.

The birth of the biotechnology industry marks the apex of drug discovery during the past two decades. The pace with which genetically engineered discoveries have moved from the lab to the clinic has been astounding. In 1975, recombinant DNA based technologies were in their infancy, and products still resided in the realm of promotional writing. In 1995, sales of products derived from recombinant DNA methods approach $8 billion–still less than 4% of total worldwide pharmaceuticals, but growing rapidly.

As a rule, seminal discoveries require intensive capital investment to take root and yield products. The biotechnology industry is no exception to this rule, but it emerged at an auspicious moment when industry, venture capitalists, and market investors were willing to bet aggressively on its future. Now, however, the drug discovery juggernaut of the past 20 years is coming face-to-face with potent counterbalancing forces, the primary one being the skyrocketing cost of getting drugs approved with marketable claims structures.

We can look at the progress of recent decades within many frames of reference. One is to consider what factors contributed to the successes of that period, and another is to look at advances in terms of truly innovative drug discoveries, value-added drug developments, and me-too agents.

## A PLAN FOR SERENDIPITY

*What we anticipate seldom occurs; what we least expected generally happens.–* Benjamin Disraeli, 1837

From time to time, serendipity tosses a winner drug in our laps. However, since the day that Alexander Fleming picked up on penicillin, the factors underlying successful drug discovery programs have generally depended less on luck and more on the combination of bright scientists and mundane benchwork. The universal goal has been to produce useful new drugs by analyzing biosystems and learning how they can be reliably influenced. To perform this function well, research directors need to marshal: (1) the ability to manipulate a desired biological target, (2) one or more relevant animal models in which to test drug candidates, and (3) some structural clue to act as a starting point for the medicinal chemists. It is rare that the aggregate of all three factors is available, but the results can be very dramatic.

A case in point has been bacteriology, where the target (bacteria) can be studied in isolation, antimicrobial activity can be examined *in vitro* and *in vivo,* and nature has offered a variety of leads for the medicinal chemist to build upon. These advantages have led to the elimination or control of many feared diseases such as pneumonia, syphilis, whooping cough, measles, and polio. The past two decades have witnessed continued successes in antimicrobial drug discovery/development, including the introduction of β-lactam and quinolone antibiotics, as well as second-, third-, and fourth-generation cephalosporins. As each new drug finds its place in therapy, the more intransigent infectious conditions become more clearly highlighted. For example, we are no further along toward curing the common cold in 1995 than we were in 1975. At the same time, we also remain plagued with such difficult to manage bacterial, fungal, and viral infections as herpes and nosocomial infections, septic shock, and AIDS.

In 1975, most drug discovery programs were heavily accented with "black box" animal models, and many engaged in broadscale screening of chemical libraries in the hope of stumbling upon the occasional diamond in the rough. Dr. Edward Paget once characterized this latter approach as "pharmacology untouched by the human mind." However, the mid-1970s found a newer and extremely powerful approach, receptor-based drug models, surging through both academe and industry. Receptor-based assays very rapidly became the norm in nearly every sector of drug discovery research. The combination of receptor-based assay systems with crystallographic techniques and receptor modeling enabled chemists–for the first time–to design lead compounds based upon receptor architecture instead of creating new leads by synthesizing variants of known drugs. The battle cry became "rational drug design," and this, in turn, has become one of the foundations of biotechnology.

The importance of receptor-driven drug discovery must not be understated, and those who employed these methods early on, such as Sir James Black in his work leading to the β-blocker propranolol and to $H_2$ antagonists (cimetidine), were regarded as giants. These were true innovator drugs, and they underscored the reality, never more true than today, that the primary path to maximum product margins runs through the valley of risky innovations. The success of the ACE inhibitors (e.g., Capoten®, Vasotec®), serotonergic antidepressants (e.g., Prozac®), and HMG-CoA reductase inhibitor hypolipidemics (e.g., Mevacor®, Pravachol®) bears further witness to this dictum.

In 1975, the debut of the NSAIDs had just taken place with Motrin®. Tagamet® was still two years from launch. The calcium channel blockers and ACE inhibitors were poised to enter the market. Cancer chemotherapy was in its infancy. Heart attack and stroke were managed by watchful waiting, and antivirals were nearly beyond conception.

TABLE 3. Diseases of the 1960s in Which Novel Pharmaceuticals Played a Central Role in Mortality Reduction.

| Diseases | Major Drugs Used to Treat |
|---|---|
| Hypertensive heart disease, hypertension | ACE inhibitors, β–blockers, $Ca^{2+}$–channel blockers, nitrates, diuretics |
| Childhood Diseases | Antibiotics, hormones, vaccines |
| Rheumatic Fever | Antibiotics |
| Peptic Ulcer | $H_2$ blockers, proton pump inhibitors |
| Emphysema | Anti-inflammatories, bronchodilators |
| Ischemic Heart Disease | ACE inhibitors, β–blockers, $Ca^{2+}$–channel blockers, thrombolytics, nitrates |

## PROGRESS IN TREATMENTS/CURES

In the period between 1975 and 1995, new pharmaceuticals offered cures for some diseases and softened the impact of many others. Hodgkin's disease, acute lymphocytic leukemia, hairy cell leukemia, and peptic ulcers became treatable conditions. Schizophrenia, depression, diabetes, angina, and congestive heart disease moved from the poorly treatable to the treatable-but-not-cured column. Control of hypertension was vastly improved, and this was paralleled by tumbling incidence rates for heart attack and stroke. Indeed, between the early 1970s and 1995, novel drug therapy has been centrally associated with profound death rate declines in many important disease categories (Table 3). Innovator drugs have saved literally millions of lives over the past two decades.

Three powerful scientific movements have been joined with progress in receptor science between 1975 and the present. The first is the biotechnology revolution, the second and third are the explosions in scientific knowledge about immunology and neuroscience.

## BIOTECH RETURN ON INVESTMENT– PROMISE OR REALITY?

The biotech industry is a compelling study in science, drug development, risk taking, and general management principles. Nearly all of the ideas informing biotechnology were original and creative. For the decade between about 1980 and 1990, the industry had that magical quality that shoots from the eyes of true believers to the wallets of investors. What is so special about biotechnology in general and recombinant DNA based R&D in particular? It is difficult to select a single overarching facet, but in terms of drug discovery, one answer is that recombinant methods generate an astonishing number of drug targets, many "arriving" with "built-in" therapeutic implications.

Among the many advantages of recombinant methods is that one can find a gene even without necessarily having identified with precision its protein product. Because DNA chemistry is vastly easier than protein chemistry, recombinant methods enable much faster isolation, identification, and replication of potentially useful bioactivities than has ever been possible in the past. The commercial result has been riveting to observe: 1,300 U.S. biotech companies, an enormous shift toward biotech programs within established pharmaceutical companies, private and public investments at the multibillion-dollar level, hundreds of lead compounds, worldwide technical races, and a blizzard of patents. Explosions are anarchic in nature, and it is therefore not surprising that the technical side of the biotech industry has often raced forward into business blunders. Again and again, technically gifted but commercially naive scientists have confused prevalence of a disease with existence of a market and activity of an agent *in vitro* with performance as a drug.

Nonetheless, the industry has produced commercially important innovator drugs such as granulocyte colony stimulating factor (Neupogen®) for oncology; erythropoietin (Epogen®) for treatment of anemia associated with renal failure, antiviral therapy, and chemotherapy; interferon (Intron A®) for treating hairy cell leukemia and improving resistance to viral infections; hepatitis B vaccine (Recombivax HB®). Indeed, the excitement surrounding recombinant products and biotech companies has been so profound that Genentech's thrombolytic drug Activase® (recombinant tissue plasminogen activator) could catalyze the expansion of interventional cardiologic methods in heart attack–in spite of the preexistence of another drug (streptokinase) of nearly equal potency.

The biotech industry has chased up many alleys, some of them blind. An example of this, at least so far, has been monoclonal antibodies. Long touted as a huge source of "magic bullets," this corner of the pharmacopeia remains sparsely populated (although in 1994, Centocor's monoclonal drug RheoPro® was the sole innovative agent approved by the FDA's Center for Biologics Research and Evaluation). At the same time, recombinant monoclonal antibodies have become a mainstay of the diagnostic industry. Because diagnostics often act as market drivers for pharmaceuticals, recombinant antigen based diagnostics must be seen as an important manifestation of the biotech revolution.

Recombinant technologies have become important not only as a source of drugs and diagnostics but also as a vital element in the R&D process. For example, recombinant methods enabled scientists to dissect the serotonin (5-HT) receptor family into several tiers of biochemical cousins (isoforms). The $5\text{-}HT_1$ receptor was characterized into four subtypes ($5\text{-}HT_1$ alpha through delta), and the delta subtype was determined to participate in setting cerebrovascular tone, thereby representing a target for antimigraine drug discovery. Once the receptor tools were developed, the first clinically useful $5\text{-}HT_{1D}$ agonist (Imigran®) soon followed.

One of the most remarkable transitions of the past 20 years has taken place in neuroscience. In 1975, the field was just coming to grips with such concepts as neurotransmitters vs. neuromodulators and small molecule chemical messengers vs. peptides. Indeed, the idea that peptides could act as essential cell-to-cell messengers in the brain was still novel, and the antibody techniques for studying such phenomena were crude. The characterization of different opioid receptors and the identification of endogenous opioid peptides (the enkephalins and endorphins) ignited a worldwide race to find one of the holy grails of neuropharmacology–a nonaddicting opioid analgesic. When the dust cleared, our molecular understanding of the brain had been advanced a generation, but no one had been able to achieve a separation between opioid-mediated analgesia and the cellular tolerance that forms the basis for addiction. Thus, not all recent scientific triumphs have enjoyed commercial expression.

Neuroscience and immunology enjoy many parallels, not the least of which is a breathtaking level of complexity. The healthy functioning brain requires the coordinated activities of billions of nerve cells, using thousands of chemical messengers to regulate trillions of connections and uncountable receptor/effector interactions. Life for the drug hunter is further complicated by the fact that it is extremely difficult to predict all of the network effects of a drug studied in isolated cells. In contrast, the immune system offers up its elements for study in the test tube but reserves the right to modulate the molecular targets of its cell surfaces constantly. The complexity of the immune system is the complexity of a near infinity of molecular configurations, all of which can be called upon to confound the drug searcher. Nonetheless, we have learned to suppress the immune system to assist with transplants and to boost the immune system to help support patients challenged by profound infection.

If we momentarily filter out the biotech revolution and look back over the past 20 years, we see a period of energetic science, a steady flow of innovative drugs and value-added drugs, insightful and clinically important advances in drug delivery (e.g., inhalers, transdermals, and controlled-release dosage forms), emergent focuses on patient compliance and quality of life issues, and excellent clinical justifications for strong product margins. When we add biotech back into the mix, we are witness to a historic scientific period, complete with early triumphs and blunders. We have been thrilled by the wonder of the biotech infant and now stand to be sobered by the demands of its adolescence.

## AND MOUNTAINS TO CLIMB

A paradox of drug discovery is that each new drug achievement in terms of disease management or cure brings greater attention to another disease, and that new disease is likely to represent an even greater pharmacological challenge than its predecessor. The 1995 list of baffling conditions is a humbling one, as shown in Table 4.

It is a second paradox that, when in the last decade enormous strides have been made in developing the molecular biological and synthetic chemistry tools to pursue the diseases that were previously beyond inspection in the lab, we should now face a tightening of regulatory and cost-containment environments that will have the inevitable effects of making product development more costly and slowing down progress. The impact is already being felt: the average industry rate of increase in R&D spending in 1994 was the slowest it has been since 1975. A corollary to this paradox is that effective pharmaceuticals reduce medical costs. The 7% pharmaceutical component of our overall health expenditure outlay helps control and reduce the 93% balance (Figure 3). Thus, in the long run, cutbacks in pharmaceutical R&D are costly to society.

## FORWARD MARCH

*Prophecy is the most gratuitous form of error.*–George Eliot, 1871

On the scientific front, the next 20 years will continue to see a flood of innovative leads from biotech (as defined broadly to include molecular biology, recombinant DNA based methodologies, receptor modeling, and many other methodologies involving the study of cell behavior). However, the cost per drug approval will continue to rise, and companies will have

TABLE 4. Remaining Untreated/Undertreated Diseases.

| | |
|---|---|
| Alzheimer's Disease | Stroke |
| Various Cancers | Macular Degeneration |
| AIDS | Periodontitis |
| Osteoporosis | Arthritis |
| Diabetes | Depression |
| Asthma | Obesity |
| Congestive Heart Disease | Parkinson's Disease |
| Schizophrenia | Diabetes |
| Multiple Sclerosis | and on and on |

FIGURE 3. Pharmaceutical Percentage of Total U.S. Health Expenditure.

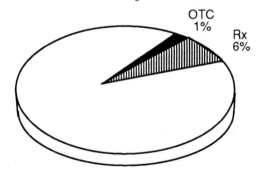

fewer and fewer options for recovering those costs. In the past, if you had to do a few more clinical trials, the cost could be recovered through the price. This is no longer an option.

R&D efforts will not, and already are not, immune to corporate consolidations. This will reduce the level of basic and applied research in the "BIGCOs," while the biotech industry is poised to experience an intense shakedown. There may be 1,300 biotech companies, but there are probably not 1,300 good ideas among them. The year 2015 will probably have witnessed many biotech company burials, a broad period of biotech company consolidation, and a slower rate of "NEWCO" formation. At the same time, the quality of new companies is likely to be much higher, on average, than was the case in the past decade. New biotech companies are unlikely to be "one-trick ponies." Instead, they will offer multiple product leads, including some broad-based "enabling" technologies. To be successful, new companies will have to have the potential to dominate in a field and to enjoy at least the possibility of straightforward development paths. Technologies will also have to offer not only the possibility of improved clinical care but also the possibility of clearly definable cost savings.

What will be seen by 2015? Some advances are just over the horizon, and we can make predictions with very limited risk. For example, there will be treatments for acute stroke, and there will be improvements in present drugs for schizophrenia, depression, migraine, and certain cancers. We have already witnessed the emergence of drug resistant microbes, and this will lend renewed urgency to the search for novel antibiotics. Will we conquer viruses? The optimist is compelled to predict progress, but one simply cannot say.

On the methodology side, the next 20 years will see combinatorial chemistry quickening the tempo of drug discovery. Carbohydrate chemistry, which has already taken tenuous root, may deliver more tangibly on its promise as basic research carries this field as close to clinical utility as it thought it was in 1990. We will also see the advent of genetic engineering, and this will have expression in actual genetic manipulations, the development of delivery vectors, and such broad areas as stem-cell manipulation and modification. As has been the case with recombinant DNA methods, gene therapy is likely to experience an explosive episode followed by a more extended interval of sobriety. Genetic manipulation is also a field that will carry with it profound ethical questions, much like a bull that carries around with it its own china shop.

Innovations will not be limited to therapeutics. For example, the recent and unexpected discovery of superconductors that can function at liquid air temperatures (the cuprates) suggests that we will see a new generation of diagnostic imaging agents (superconducting quantum interference devices, or SQUIDs) that are more powerful and, possibly, less harmful than presently available imaging methods.

The overall pace of discovery will certainly be slowed by cost pressures, but the appearance of a few innovative and commercially high-profile drugs might greatly reduce the resistance to investment. A difficult barrier, at least in the U.S., will be the FDA, which continues to clear about 24 new drugs per year (a rate largely unchanged since 1975). User fees will help, but nothing short of a sea change in the drug review process will alter the present regulatory bottleneck.

The challenge between now and 2015 may be, indeed, to learn how to better manage high-risk research so that it may continue to feed development pipelines with innovative drugs. Drug leads will have to be developed under a more deferred risk structure than has been the case in the past. Another way to say this is that technology transfer must become less front-end loaded. Distribution of wealth will follow more from product sales and less from the promise of potential product sales. Overall, perhaps the best news is that the tide of innovative drugs promises to offer clinically important advances for the patient and the possibility of sustained growth for the industry as a whole.

### MATURITY? EXCELLENCE?

*It takes a long time to bring excellence to maturity.* – Publius Syrus Maxum, 780.

Is the pharmaceutical industry mature? Certainly not yet in 1995; perhaps so by 2015–if society can afford continued progress. We're still a growth industry for the next 20 years, certainly by comparison to other industries.

If not mature, then are we enjoying excellence? If that standard is defined by whether we make people's lives better, the answer is yes. If defined by whether we are building shareholder value, again in the affirmative. If defined by our constant innovation, yes, again! If defined by whether we are efficient, the answer is increasingly positive.

Perhaps all we need is 20 more years of excellence to reach maturity.

# The Influence
# of Pharmaceutical Technology
# on Marketing New Drugs
# and Optimizing Therapeutic Outcomes

### David W. Newton

*New drug delivery systems . . . will replace traditional drug therapy. Many will require new expertise and new services. (1)*

## INTRODUCTION

### The Drug Therapy Outcomes
### to Delivery Systems Connection

Contemporary therapeutic outcomes research is vital to the professional survival and advancement of practicing pharmacists, whether or not they know it. The goal is to prove that direct and indirect patient care services by pharmacists result in patients' increased life and health quality for a lower economic cost than would occur without pharmaceutical care by pharmacists.

It is likely, but still to be decisively documented, that controlled drug

---

David W. Newton, Ph.D., is Professor and Chairman in the Department of Pharmaceutics, Albany College of Pharmacy, 106 New Scotland Avenue, Albany, NY 12208-3492.

[Haworth co-indexing entry note]: "The Influence of Pharmaceutical Technology on Marketing New Drugs and Optimizing Therapeutic Outcomes." Newton, David W. Co-published simultaneously in *Journal of Pharmaceutical Marketing & Management* (Pharmaceutical Products Press, an imprint of The Haworth Press, Inc.) Vol. 10, No. 2/3, 1996, pp. 19-29; and *Pharmaceutical Marketing in the 21st Century* (ed: Mickey C. Smith): Pharmaceutical Products Press, an imprint of The Haworth Press, Inc., 1996, pp. 19-29. Single or multiple copies of this article are available from The Haworth Document Delivery Service [1-800-342-9678, 9:00 a.m. - 5:00 p.m. (EST)].

delivery technologies are an increasingly valuable therapeutic tool in the foregoing mission (2). For example, the virtually infallible performance of transdermal patches allows marketing of fentanyl, nicotine, and scopolamine in unit-of-use dosages so dangerously large that they would not be approved in traditional dosage forms for self-administration by patients.

### The Well-Kept Secret of Pharmaceutical Technology

Both within and outside the health care professions, pharmaceutical technology probably connotes drug chemicals more than finished drug products. However, pharmacists know that pharmaceutical technology means the ingredients, conditions, and processes of manufacturing, or compounding, and the mechanisms and measures of drug release from formulations that are used to administer drugs clinically.

Unlike the case for drug chemicals, the value of specific pharmaceutical technologies per se has either not been researched or the research results have not been published. This observation seems well illustrated in the appraisal by Sir James Black (JB), the 1988 Nobel laureate in medicine whose premier contribution was the pharmacological development of propranolol. The following comments are from a late 1988 interview of Black by the journal *Pharmaceutical Technology* (PT) (3):

PT:    . . . the public is frequently critical of the pharmaceutical industry. What can be done to rectify the situation?

JB:    I think both the press and industry have failed to communicate to the public that behind every little pill is a vast amount of high technology. It really is incredibly complex, but to the public a pill looks very simple.

If "pills" (powder-filled capsules and compressed tablets) are "incredibly complex," then what does that say for osmotic tablets and transdermal patches? Pharmacists also know the answer to this, and, because of the less frequent and more comfortable use of the latter two, the public thinks they are even *simpler.*

### A So-Obvious-It-Is-Ignored Case: Generic Equivalent Drugs

Generic equivalent drugs are the most prominent evidence of the therapeutic–thus, economic–value of pharmaceutical formulations, independent of the drug chemicals they deliver. Marketing approval of generics by the U.S. Food and Drug Administration is really for their precisely reproducible pharmaceutical technology. That technology enables generics to provide practically the same rate and extent of systemic drug absorption as the original brand-name drug products against which they are judged. Finally, of course, measured bioequivalency is presumed to equal clinical equivalency.

## POST-1970s ADVANCES
## IN PHARMACEUTICAL TECHNOLOGY

### Drug Delivery Systems versus Dosage Forms

The period from 1940 to 1970 has been called the physical pharmacy age in both pharmacy education and industry (4). The 1968 founding of the ALZA Corporation led within a decade to pharmaceutical scientists disagreeing over how to describe the historically unique domain of pharmacy, namely, products to put drugs into and onto the body (5, 6).

The ALZA Corporation pioneered constant release rate transdermal patches and osmotic tablets, which publicly symbolize the stark difference between controlled drug delivery systems and traditional drug dosage forms. There is no longer, nor did it last long, any semantic rift over those two terminologies for the technologies they represent.

### Why Are Delivery Systems Novel and Controlled?

Conventional dosage forms contain drugs simply as a uniform physical mixture. Typically, most or all of the entire dose is available for release *in vivo* at the same time after it is administered. However, high variability of gastrointestinal events for swallowed drugs, especially those in solid form, results in relatively large variability in the times and heights of peak concentrations in plasma.

Drug release from controlled delivery systems is predetermined by an integral mechanism or structure. That control system generally accounts for physiological effects that would otherwise cause inconsistent or inadequate plasma concentration versus time profiles. The word novel connotes innovations such as nearly constant-rate absorption rate from transdermal patches and osmotic pressure-pumped tablets. Controlled describes a precise rate, extent, timing, or location (targeting) of drug delivery *in vivo*.

### Renaissance in Pharmaceutical Technology: ca 1980

Since 1900, predicting patient response to drug therapy has evolved from being based on (1) the name of pharmacist-compounded medications of vastly different potency to (2) a precise amount of pure drug administered in standardized dosage forms to (3) drug in plasma monitoring to (4) rate, time, and space control of drug delivery in the body.

Pharmaceutical technology was revolutionized with ALZA's Transderm-Scop® patch in 1981 and Eli Lilly & Co.'s Humulin® recombinant DNA insulin in 1982. Those pioneer products have been followed by rapid and intensely competitive innovation in an industry seemingly content since the 1940s with gradually improving synthetic drug chemicals and status quo dosage forms.

## THE POTENTIAL ECONOMIC IMPACT OF PHARMACEUTICAL TECHNOLOGY PER SE

### Apparent Public Expectations of Pharmaceutical Technology

Americans seem to expect access to the most recent drug therapy advances as if access were a Bill of Rights entitlement. In 1994, eight biotechnology or genetically engineered protein drugs approved since 1985 by the FDA consumed 10% of nonfederal hospitals' annual drug budgets, each of which must pay for hundreds of individual drugs (7). A dilemma looms as public demand for more costly and effective drugs rises, while payment to those prescribing and dispensing them does not keep pace. The convenience and predictable good performance of controlled pharmaceutical delivery technologies is also increasingly expected.

### Predicted Economic Growth of Controlled Drug Delivery Market

A 1992 forecast for U.S. sales of controlled and targeted drug delivery systems shows a rise from $445 million in 1990 to $2.1 billion by 1997 (Figure 1) (8). Approximately 15% of the predicted annual growth is for parenteral infusion devices, which are not drug-specific, integrated delivery systems.

### Can Delivery Technologies Be Separately Valued?

The data in Figure 1 do not represent the "empty" delivery technologies, i.e., they do not refer to liposomes and transdermal patches *without* drugs. That is because the clinical pharmaceutical performance of controlled and targeted delivery systems results from the intimate integration, or interdependency, of the drug chemical and the other components, ingredients, and mechanisms. For example, it is simple to assign a cost to empty two-piece hard gelatin capsules. However, it is not so easy, if possible at all, to evaluate the economic and health influence of that capsule shell on patient outcomes of drug therapy.

It seems that a more relevant and achievable objective would be to analyze the human and economic values of therapy with controlled drug delivery technologies versus traditional dosage forms of the same or equivalent drug chemicals. The perceived therapeutic value of "pharmaceutical technology is analogous to that of starring actors in a successful play depending on so-obvious-they-are-taken-for-granted good props" (9).

## The Drug Chemicals in the Future Delivery Systems

The drug chemicals now in FDA-approved controlled delivery systems, such as transdermal patches, are not themselves new. In fact, several are pre-1962 drugs, which means that (a) they were not subject to the placebo-controlled clinical testing requirements of the 1962 Harris-Kefauver new

FIGURE 1. U.S. Sales of Alternative Drug Delivery Systems.*

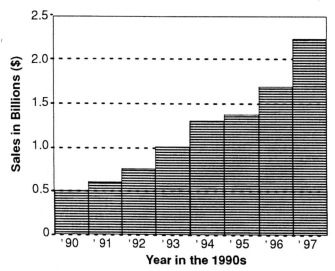

*Adapted from Weintraub M. The alternative drug delivery systems market. P&T 1992;17:167.

drug application amendment to the original 1938 U.S. Food, Drug and Cosmetic Act and (b) they are generally recognized as safe and effective based on their historic uses and dosage regimens.

During the next two decades, a variety of increasingly convenient and versatile controlled and targeted drug delivery technologies will be marketed to deliver both old natural and synthetic drugs and new biotechnology drugs. Scores of promising biotechnology drug chemicals are being tested in humans, and still more are under preclinical research (7, 10, 11).

Most of the investment cost of a new drug (i.e., new according to FDA regulations and definition) is for premarketing clinical trials, not for preclinical pharmaceutical development. Yet, for an increasing number of new drugs, the chemical and its delivery technology or system are inseparably codependent for FDA approval.

While it is predicted that protein drugs will continue to grow in pharmacologic–and thus economic–value, there are still three inherent problems with them (7-12). First, because proteins are either erratically absorbed or metabolically inactivated when swallowed, they are now administered by patient-*un*friendly injection. Second, proteins are generally unstable and reactive. Third, many proteins have a relatively short residence in plasma after injection. Therefore, specialized, more patient-friendly technologies to deliver proteins are vital to the future marketing success of proteins, especially in a growing population of very sick people treated in their homes (12-15).

### Controlled Delivery Systems and Pharmacy Dispensing Practice

For decades, pharmacists have expected weekly or monthly sales of insulin products to some patients for years. However, technology is advancing such that during the next ten years subcutaneous insulin injections may be replaced. It is challenging to predict the impact on pharmacy dispensing of insulin administered via nasal sprays and oral delivery systems, self-regulated implants, artificial pancreases with monoclonal insulin-producing cells, and genetically engineered immunomodulating proteins that prevent or cure diabetes.

Except in cases when the drug chemical has an intrinsic action or elimination half-life of more than 24 hours, nearly all traditional dosage forms, which contain drug dosages in milligrams, are administered 1 or more times daily. Current and future biotechnology protein drug doses are measured in micrograms, nanograms, and even smaller portions. Therefore, they can be administered from very small controlled delivery systems over days, months, or years of action per single unit or refilling.

## In Vivo *Drug Targeting: The* In Vivo *Space Frontier*

What might be the dollar market value of delivery technologies that would deliver a drug only to a selected body site, organ, or cell type? Imagine, for example, gentamicin only in cells infected with susceptible bacteria and not in the systemic bloodstream. Even with the best pharmacokinetic monitoring, conventional intravenous gentamicin solution therapy can cause renal failure and ototoxicity and result in therapeutic failure. Surely the higher acquisition expense of targeted *in vivo* delivery products such as liposomes would be less than the human suffering and economic cost of gentamicin toxicities and inadequate therapeutic response.

Intravenous liposomes, among other novel technologies, hold promise for effective targeted drug delivery. They are microscopic fluid vesicles similar to mammalian cell membranes. In clinical trials, liposomes of amphotericin B, doxorubicin, and gentamicin have improved therapy and lowered toxicity compared to solutions.

Current liposomes target some afflicted and infected tissue sites because the latter contain a high density of blood-cleaning macrophages. Labeling liposomes with antibodies or surface reactive chemicals will lead to more tissue-selective delivery.

### *Dosage Exposure Timing Control: Chronotherapeutics*

Usually, the total daily dosage of drugs is administered either (1) in a temporally symmetrical time pattern (i.e., 1 dosage portion every 4 to 24 hours) or (2) continuously (constant delivery rate infusions, osmotic tablets, and transdermal patches). Such arbitrary temporal patterns produce either (1) repeating series of peaks and troughs or (2) a relatively invariable or constant drug in plasma concentration. Both of those patterns usually ignore the recurrent rhythms of biological drug-related events, i.e., chronotherapy (16).

Chronotherapeutics is the study and practice of timing drug exposure to cause maximum health benefit and minimum harm from drug therapy. Controlled drug delivery systems offer the advantage of temporal adjustability of dosage exposure in synchrony with drug-related biological rhythms of pharmacologic, pharmacokinetic, cytokinetic, endocrine, and enzymatic processes. It already has valuable, yet not widely respected or adopted, application to therapy of asthma, gastroesophageal reflux disease, and cancer (16).

## *CONCLUSION*

Compared to traditional dosage forms, controlled delivery technologies can, or will, precisely regulate the *in vivo* site, timing, and extent of drug exposure. The marketing success of such advanced pharmaceutical products will require that their higher acquisition costs be fairly evaluated. For example, the cost of lifetime treatable adverse effects and clinical failures resulting from traditional bolus release capsules and tablets to treat asthma could make one nightly osmotic tablet, costing many times more each, a bargain. The economic savings from, i.e., the marketing incentive for, controlled drug delivery technologies result from the following gains in patient care outcomes from drug therapy:

1. Reduce lifetime drug dosage exposure during chronic therapy, for example, transdermal estradiol compared to conjugated estrogen tablets
2. Enable chronotherapy to maximize the benefit and minimize the harm from drug therapy
3. Minimize or avoid the influence of gastrointestinal physiological and dietary effects on oral drug bioavailability
4. Maintain a precise narrow range, or specific value, of drug in plasma concentrations, thus improving therapeutic responses with fewer distressing and treatable adverse effects
5. Reduce the frequency and increase the convenience of drug administration, which increases patient compliance
6. Function by dependable integral mechanisms that prevent bolus release of potentially dangerous dosages contained in one long-acting unit.

Various delivery system technologies are under investigation to customize therapy according to the patient and the diagnosis. Tables 1 and 2 list some examples, applications, and advantages of administration route specific controlled drug delivery systems (13, 14, 17, 18). What can be expected from their FDA marketing approval is suggested by the following comment: "Transdermals, predicted . . . in the 1960s, have now become a billion-dollar market and added financial incentives to investigation" (19).

TABLE 1. Body Access Routes and Types or Mechanisms of Some Novel Controlled Drug Delivery Systems.

## Intravenous Injection

- o/w microemulsions [nonionized drug in oil microdrops]
- liposome phospholipid vesicles
- external magnet-targetable microspheres
- tissue or cell targeted drug + macromolecule or monoclonal antibody [mAb] complexes
- slow releasing drug + biopolymer microparticles
- cyclodextrin-solubilized hydrophobic drugs in water
- prodrugs that cross the blood brain barrier to be converted by enzymes and "trapped" or targeted as more polar molecules

## Oral Ingestion

- geometric, gel structure, and osmotic pressure controlled drug release from tablets
- bioadhesive excipients to regionalize intestinal absorption
- enzyme-inhibitors reduce intestinal and first-pass metabolism
- electronically monitored and regulated solution-filled capsules
- constant-release osmotic pressure devices loaded with layers of drug and excipients to control the time of release relative to the time of ingestion

## Subdermal Tissue Implants and Injections

- biopolymer membrane surrounded systems that release proteins and small molecules via (a) chemical or enzymatic reaction, (b) dissolution, diffusion, erosion, or expansion and contraction, (c) magnetic force, and (d) ultrasound or phonophoresis

## Transdermal Flux

- wearable devices regulated by (a) direct current iontophoresis [drug ion flow) and electro-osmosis [drug solution flow], (b) laser beam, (c) magnetic force, and (d) ultrasound
- plain and chemically enhanced diffusion from patches

## Transmucosal Flux

- films, gels, liposomes, and sprays for inhalation and application to mucous membranes

TABLE 2. Prospective Clinical Advantages of Some Controlled Drug Delivery Systems Over Conventional Dosage Forms.

| Novel Controlled | Comparative Conventional Dosage Form | Advantages of Delivery System[a] |
|---|---|---|
| IV liposomes | IV solution | High targeted tissue or cell and low (nontoxic) plasma concentration; isotonic |
| IV microemulsion | IV solution | Lower (nontoxic) maximum and longer effective plasma concentration; isotonic |
| Biopolymer tissue implants | injections; PO solids | Safe, prolonged, and time and dose variable plasma concentrations |
| Inhaled liposomes | inhaled mists and powders; injections | Higher pulmonary intracellular concentration with lower systemic exposure |
| Intranasal sprays | injections | Noninvasive; lower effective dosage; less traumatic; safer |
| Osmotic tablets | PO solids and fluids | Physiologically unperturbed release rate and time; once daily or real time initiated dosage |
| PO solids with bioadhesives or enzyme inhibitors | PO solids and fluids; injections | Precise bioavailability; adequate peptide and protein absorption |
| Transdermal patches | SL injections and PO tablets | Chronic lower plasma concentration; avoid extreme peak and trough plasma concentrations; lower lifetime dosage |

[a]IV is intravenous; PO is per oral or via ingestion; SL is sublingual.

# REFERENCES

1. Hepler CD. Unresolved issues in the future of pharmacy. Am J Hosp Pharm 1988;45:1071-81.

2. Giorgianni SJ. "Dosage form" definition may limit generic use. NABP Newsl 1994;23(9):116.

3. Schuber S. An interview with Sir James Black. Pharm Tech 1989;13(3):48+.

4. Hepler CD. The third wave in pharmaceutical education: the clinical movement. Am J Pharm Educ 1987;51:369-85.

5. Benson H, Mader W. Drug dosage forms. J Pharm Sci 1977;66:VIII.

6. Chien YW, Robinson JR. "Smart" drug-delivery systems. J Parenter Sci Technol 1982;36:231.

7. Santell JP. Projecting future drug expenditures-1995. Am J Health-Syst Pharm 1995;52:151-63.

8. Weintraub M. The alternative drug delivery systems market. P&T 1992;17:167.

9. Newton DW. Pharmaceutical technology and drug therapy outcomes. APhA-APRS Acad Reporter 1995;3(1):in press.

10. Johnson NE. Pharmacoeconomics and biotech drugs. P&T 1992;17:1402-12.

11. Dibner MD. U.S. biotechnology and pharmaceuticals. BioPharm 1992;5(8):24-8.

12. Ratafia M. Drug delivery: the key to biotechnology markets. Med Market Media 1989;24(Oct 1):11-21.

13. Langer R. New methods of drug delivery. Science 1990;249:1527-33.

14. Robinson DH, Mauger JW. Drug delivery systems. Am J Hosp Pharm 1991;48 (Suppl 1):S14-S23.

15. Piascik MM. Research and development of drugs and biologic entities. Am J Hosp Pharm 1991;48(Suppl 1):S4-S13.

16. Traynor K, Newton DW, Hrushesky WJM, Reiter RJ. A pharmacist's primer on chronotherapeutics. Am Pharm 1992;NS32:261-9.

17. Newton DW. Prospects for controlled-delivery systems. Am Pharm 1992;NS32: 989- 93.

18. Newton DW. Biotechnology and controlled drug delivery. US Pharm 1991;16 (6):38+.

19. Maibach HI. Review of *Skin Permeation Fundamentals and Application*. J Pharm Sci 1994;83:1524.

# Marketing Medicines for Self-Medication

## Jerome A. Reinstein

### INTRODUCTION

There is a worldwide trend for people to take greater charge of their own health. The World Health Organization stated this was a desirable trend in the Alma-Ata Declaration in 1978 which endorsed the goal of health for all by the year 2000, with primary health care being the key to attaining it. It stated, *inter alia,* that "the people have the right and duty to participate individually and collectively in the planning and implementation of their health care" (1). Subsequently, WHO's *Guidelines for Developing National Drug Policies,* in its chapter on self-medication, stated that "it is desirable to encourage self-medication and every attempt should be made to ensure its appropriate use and to guard against any unacceptable risks it may entail" (2). Independent studies of self-medication habits and practices in 14 countries have demonstrated that consumers generally do use nonprescription medicines responsibly and safely (3).

Primary health care has a somewhat different meaning in different cultural/economic contexts. In the developing countries, it can refer to centers in rural areas which may be staffed by nonmedical health personnel. In developed countries, it may refer to care before medical intervention and also to a general practitioner (GP). In any event, responsible self-medication forms an important part of primary health care, as the individual is the first person to recognize minor health problems and, with sufficient education and information, can successfully treat these problems

Jerome A. Reinstein, Ph.D., is an industry consultant and Director-General of the World Federation of Proprietary Medicine Manufacturers, 15 Sydney House, Woodstock Road, London W4 1DP, U.K.

[Haworth co-indexing entry note]: "Marketing Medicines for Self-Medication." Reinstein, Jerome A. Co-published simultaneously in *Journal of Pharmaceutical Marketing & Management* (Pharmaceutical Products Press, an imprint of The Haworth Press, Inc.) Vol. 10, No. 2/3, 1996, pp. 31-38; and: *Pharmaceutical Marketing in the 21st Century* (ed: Mickey C. Smith) Pharmaceutical Products Press, an imprint of The Haworth Press, Inc., 1996, pp. 31-38. Single or multiple copies of this article are available from The Haworth Document Delivery Service [1-800-342-9678, 9:00 a.m. - 5:00 p.m. (EST)].

without referral to the medical system. Self-medication is now recognized as an important part of the total health care system.

Responsible self-medication may be defined as the rational use of medicines designed, labeled, and authorized for self-care. Self-medication itself is as old as humanity. Since primitive times, people have cared for their own health using what was in nature around them to help cure or alleviate their ailments. Use of plant-derived medicines, especially, continues to this day. It is much stronger in some countries than in others, but everywhere some plant medicines are still used, and many active ingredients of others are still to be discovered.

It is largely since 1945, however, that the self-medication field as a separate industry has really come into its own, although proprietary associations have existed for over 100 years in North America. Initially, most countries required only that nonprescription medicines be safe, leaving efficacy to be determined by the marketplace. The assumption was that if a medicine did no harm, the consumer could judge whether it was effective.

Over the last 30 years, governments have added efficacy as a required characteristic as well, and now most countries in the world require acceptable quality, safety, and efficacy for all medicines to be on the market legally. But what constitutes safety with self-medication? Safety is always relative: nothing, even water, is 100% safe if taken in excess. So judgments must be made to determine whether a medicinal product is safe enough to be used without professional supervision.

As the science of pharmacovigilance (drug safety monitoring) develops, we are able to determine more accurately and more quickly whether medicines cause significant problems in use. This allows us to determine that many medicines originally on prescription have a sufficiently good safety profile in use to allow them to be available without prescription for certain self-recognizable indications.

All people of the world take some medicines by self-medication, and in many countries, the differentiation between prescription medicines and nonprescription medicines is not clear or is even nonexistent. Even where there is a legal distinction between medicines that are restricted to prescription and those that may be purchased without prescription, in most countries outside of North America, Europe, and Australia, many medicines that are supposed to be restricted to prescription can be purchased without a prescription. This means that self-medication takes on a broader meaning for authorities in these countries. The responsible self-medication industry insists on distinguishing between products that are designed, tested, labeled, evaluated, and approved for self-medication and those medicines that should be used under medical supervision but are sometimes purchased without a prescription. This can be called "self-prescription" or "under-the-counter medicines" and should not be confused with true OTC medicines.

The last 50 years have seen the rapid and dramatic development of government-sponsored health care. Each country has developed ways of supplying health care to its people. Some supply most health care free through government health services or social security systems, while many supply at least some health care either free or with some contribution from the public. State-supported health care has been running into more and more budget problems in the last 20 years for a number of reasons: expectations have increased; the populations are aging, requiring more care; medical technology has developed important new diagnostic and treatment tools which frequently are very expensive; and new medicines that are more effective and safer, while prolonging life, are also expensive to develop. Along with governments' awareness of the impossibility of continuing to pay for all medical care has been an increasing desire on the part of the public for more self-reliance in health care. In many countries immediately after World War II, particularly in Europe, government policies tended to encourage people to be dependent on the state for all health care (4). Governments are now trying to wean their citizens away from total reliance on the state for health care and are encouraging people to take care of themselves when this is appropriate.

## THE PRESCRIPTION-TO-OTC SWITCH

How is it that a medicine available one day only by prescription can suddenly be released for self-medication safely? Some pharmacists ask this question. The answer is that pharmacovigilance studies over many years of marketing of the medicine at a particular dose (or higher) for certain indications assure that unsupervised use with proper labeling will be safe. The number of medicines being switched from prescription-only sale to nonprescription sale has increased markedly over the last few years. While the switch process is still rather slow in the United States and in most other countries, the U.K. has taken the lead in developing a procedure worked out in agreement among government, pharmacists, and industry that allows the evaluation of the switch request to take place within one year. Thus, some two dozen products have been switched in the last two years with this new procedure. Ingredients that some time ago would have been thought unsuitable for self-medication are proving popular with consumers and are safe for their use, given the right dose and indications. These include the $H_2$ antagonists such as cimetidine, famotidine, and ranitidine in lower dose specifically for heartburn and acid indigestion, but not for ulcer. (As of this writing, the Nonprescription Drugs Advisory Committee of the FDA has just recommended the switch of cimetidine in the U.S.) These medicines have an advantage over antacids in that their duration of action is much longer, which allows them to prevent even nighttime heartburn. One of the most effective treatments for seasonal rhinitis is topical application of very low-dose potent steroids. Beclomethasone is probably the most well-known one. It has recently been switched in nose spray form to nonprescription use in the U.K., as has flunisolide. Switching of potent steroids a few years ago was not considered feasible.

## TRADE NAMES

Should nonprescription medicines be allowed to be marketed with the same trade name (or a related name) as their prescription medicine counterparts? While a number of countries feel this could cause safety problems, those that do allow it have found that there is little, if any, confusion among either pharmacists or the public and that, on the contrary, the use of a known name allows both the pharmacist and the public to take advantage of the newly switched product more quickly. Another fear in some countries is that allowing similar names will cause an increase in requests for the prescription medication. In countries where prescription medications are fully or partially reimbursed, this could increase the social security costs. But two recent examples suggest that this is not the case. Neither the $H_2$ antagonists nor Zovirax®, when switched, produced increases in prescriptions, whereas nonprescription use of Zovirax cream for cold sores increased fivefold. This is not surprising when one considers that the drug was a major advance in the treatment of this nuisance ailment. Zovirax in an oral form for genital herpes has been considered in the United States for OTC status but has not yet been approved.

## DISTRIBUTION

Countries differ with regard to where nonprescription medicines may be sold. In many countries, they are restricted to pharmacies, even though in some of these countries a pharmacist is not always present. In others, some medicines are restricted to pharmacy while others may be sold outside of pharmacy. In still others, such as the United States, all nonprescription medicines may be sold in any outlet. The reasoning is that if it is safe enough to be used in self-medication, the labeling is adequate to assure safe and effective use. In cultures where the pharmacist has a long tradition of a monopoly on medicines, such as in a majority of the countries of the European Union (EU), all medicines are restricted to sale in a pharmacy. This is now being challenged in some countries, and we may soon see a change. Although the argument for keeping all medicines in a pharmacy for possible supervision of the sale by a pharmacist makes some theoretical sense, in practice it has not been shown that sale outside of a pharmacy is detrimental to public health.

## *ADVERTISING*

Along with distribution, one must consider advertising and promotion of nonprescription medicines. In most countries of the world, such advertising to the public of medicines that are legally available without prescription is permitted. In most countries, advertising is also controlled through strict laws, self-regulation by the industry, or, more often, a combination of the two. In fact, the self-medication industry has its own guidelines for national codes of advertising practice which, through WFPMM, it recommends to all of its member associations and companies. All companies now have their own strict review and appraisal of advertising. The combination of company self-discipline, industry self-regulation, and government law controls the advertising of nonprescription medicines. Consumer organizations and others have the role of criticizing and complaining when they feel that the advertising is not appropriate; this is done through studies and channels that have been set up. The fact that there are very few complaints and even fewer that have been upheld by advertising standards authorities suggests that OTC advertising controls are effective.

What can advertising do and not do? Many who are not in the industry or in the advertising field do not appreciate that advertising has certain built-in limitations for effectively communicating information. Advertising is a low-involvement medium. Several independent research studies have demonstrated that advertising to the public is not an effective or suitable means for communicating detailed information on the use of medicines (5, 6). Many OTC advertisements are in the form of 30-second television commercials in which only a very limited amount of information can be effectively communicated. This information includes the name of the product, what it can be used for, and a specific indication to always read the label or to follow the directions. The consumer who is tempted to determine whether he or she should buy the product as a result of advertising or other recommendations should be able to handle the package and determine from the label whether the product is suitable for the specific use in mind. Once the product is purchased and before use, the label and/or the leaflet should give more specific instructions on dosage and how to take the product.

Interestingly, until the European directive on medicine labels and leaflets came into force in 1994, OTC medicines in most European countries where medicines are restricted to sale in pharmacies and are not on self-selection had very little on the label other than the contents and the expiration date. Now they are also required to have the instructions for use of the product and any necessary warnings (7). Most medicines, including OTC medicines, have leaflets in most European countries, and eventually, all medicines will have them in European Union countries because the additional required information is so extensive that it would be difficult to print on an ordinary size label. The requirements are uniform now throughout the EU for what information should be on the label and in the leaflet.

## CONSEQUENCES FOR PHARMACISTS, PHYSICIANS, AND CONSUMERS

Pharmacists should welcome an increased number of medicines available for self-medication, as they are frequently the first port of call and would need to apply their professional knowledge more frequently to counsel consumers about the medicines. This enhances their professional status. Also, the advertising brings people into the pharmacy, where customers may discover other items they need.

Doctors are frequently hesitant to recommend OTCs in many countries because they feel that the person who comes to see them or consults with them is automatically a patient, even if all the person needs is the equivalent of an OTC medicine. But some GPs realize that they should be encouraging people to take care of their own minor illnesses rather than occupying physician time. These physicians recognize that good OTC medicines can be important in improving the quality of life of their patients when it is not necessary to have a medical visit.

Consumers and consumer organizations are looking for empowerment and choice. The UN Charter on Consumer Protection lists five rights of the consumer (Figure 1). Within the right of choice one must know what is available, and this is where advertising is important and necessary. Also, advertising is important for competition, which gives wider choice to consumers. Consumers know that they can save time and money by using appropriate OTC medicines rather than visiting the doctor and getting a

FIGURE 1. United Nations Charter on Consumer Protection.

```
┌─────────────────────────────────────┐
│                                     │
│        UNITED NATIONS CHARTER       │
│       ON CONSUMER PROTECTION        │
│                                     │
│      FIVE BASIC CONSUMER RIGHTS     │
│                                     │
│              Access                 │
│              Choice                 │
│            Information              │
│              Redress                │
│               Safety                │
│                                     │
└─────────────────────────────────────┘
```

prescription for a minor ailment. Of course, in countries where consumers get "free" medical care and "free" prescriptions, unless the time element is important, it is more difficult to convince consumers to spend their own money for medicines. But even in those countries this is happening increasingly as more effective ingredients are released for OTC sale for new indications.

## WHO RECOGNITION OF SELF-MEDICATION

The World Health Organization has recognized self-medication as a separate domain from prescription medicines by according the status of Nongovernmental Organization in Official Relations with WHO to the World Federation of Proprietary Medicine Manufacturers (WFPMM) as representing the worldwide self-medication industry. In this function, WFPMM participates in all relevant Expert Committee Meetings and contributes to WHO projects within its area of expertise.

## SELF-MEDICATION: DEVELOPING COUNTRIES vs. DEVELOPED COUNTRIES

Should self-medication be different in developing countries than it is in developed countries? In developing countries, where people generally have less money to spend on health and the governments are less able to give full health coverage, reliable self-medication products are particularly important in improving quality of life. Needless to say, inappropriate self-medication, such as the use of antibiotics when the specific illness has not been properly diagnosed, should be discouraged, and educational efforts should be made so that, for example, parents can distinguish between a cold and potential pneumonia requiring immediate treatment by a health practitioner.

In summary, responsible self-medication increases self-reliance in health and improves the quality of life for consumers while helping government control health care costs.

## REFERENCES

1. Alma-Ata 1978: primary health care. Report of the International Conference on Primary Health Care, Alma-Ata, USSR, September 6-12, 1978. Geneva: World Health Organization, 1978.

2. World Health Organization. Guidelines for developing national drug policies. Geneva: World Health Organization, 1988.

3. Reinstein J. Worldwide studies on self-medication: what do they show? Swiss Pharma 1991;13(11a):21-5.

4. Nakajima H. WFPMM 9th General Assembly Keynote Address. Swiss Pharma 1989;11(11a):14-6.

5. Taylor Nelson Research. Information or communication? A consumer study of television advertising. London: Taylor Nelson Research, 1990.

6. Kepplinger HM. How far can advertising be used to inform? Swiss Pharma 1990;12(5a):73-7.

7. Official Journal of the European Communities. No. L 113/8. 30.04.92. Council Directive 92/27/EEC of 31 March 1992. On the labelling of medicinal products for human use and on package leaflets.

# Research Databases
# for Postmillennium Health Care

Basya Gale
Paul Smith
Paul Wilson

## *INTRODUCTION*

As with Nietzsche's abyss, the pharmaceutical industry of today stares into the millennium, and the millennium stares back (maybe because there are so many new faces in it). The assumption that frightens the industry, of course, is that health care after the year 2000 will be so strange and new that the marketing and selling tools and techniques that we, as an industry, have created and to some degree mastered will be of no value to us. The perspective of this article is not so bleak. We do not expect to be looking at a world in which industry goals are no longer recognizable or achievable. Nor do we expect that all of our research and marketing tools will be without value. There will be, of course, some new terrain: new customers that the pharmaceutical industry has not addressed before and perhaps a new set of needs to go with them. Understandably, new customers make marketers nervous because marketing can no longer rely on gut instinct to make decisions. However, the pharmaceutical industry can turn to well-developed marketing research resources (both primary and secondary) which can provide the information marketers need.

Basya Gale, Ph.D., is Marketing Group Director, New Product Development; Paul Smith is Director, Statistical Services; and Paul Wilson is Vice President, Statistical Services, all at IMS America, 660 W. Germantown Pike, Plymouth Meeting, PA 19462-0905.

[Haworth co-indexing entry note]: "Research Databases for Postmillennium Health Care." Gale, Basya, Paul Smith, and Paul Wilson. Co-published simultaneously in *Journal of Pharmaceutical Marketing & Management* (Pharmaceutical Products Press, an imprint of The Haworth Press, Inc.) Vol. 10, No. 2/3, 1996, pp. 39-59; and: *Pharmaceutical Marketing in the 21st Century* (ed: Mickey C. Smith) Pharmaceutical Products Press, an imprint of The Haworth Press, Inc., 1996, pp. 39-59. Single or multiple copies of this article are available from The Haworth Document Delivery Service [1-800-342-9678, 9:00 a.m. - 5:00 p.m. (EST)].

Our view is that pharmaceutical marketing will not be so radically different in the new millennium. Marketers will still need to understand who their customers are, what the customers want, and how to configure products and services to meet those needs. Pharmaceutical industry marketers will still look to the four P's of marketing to manage their brands. What may change are the specifics, i.e., which of the four P's is most important and to which customer or customer type. What won't change is the availability of marketing tools to manage the business. Instead, tools may become both more sophisticated and more accessible.

To support this reassuring argument, we will review briefly the present resources that pharmaceutical marketers have for understanding their health care customers' needs and how marketers use these resources today. We will then explore three possible future health care industry scenarios and the customers (new and old) and customer needs generated by each scenario. Finally, we will propose adaptations and extensions of secondary research resources that might be required under each scenario (including both new information and new information management tools), and we will discuss the ways in which these resources might be used to achieve health care marketers' future goals.

## PHARMACEUTICAL MARKETERS' RESOURCES AND THEIR USES TODAY

Pharmaceutical marketers' primary goal for the past 30 years or more has been to meet their *physician* customers' needs for innovative products to treat both chronic and acute diseases and to provide continuous improvement in patients' quality and quantity of life. They have successfully met these goals, in good part as a result of rich databases that define these customer needs at the finest level and measure industry achievement and dynamics with great sensitivity.

For well over 30 years, the pharmaceutical industry has been enriched by the availability of comprehensive, ongoing marketing research databases which track market size and market dynamics at both macro and micro levels. Supporting today's pharmaceutical and health care marketing decisions are ongoing monthly (in some cases, weekly) audits of market sales (at a virtual census level) by channel of distribution, retail market prescriptions by prescriber and outlet, medical diagnosis and treatment decisions by geographic and patient and physician demographic segments, promotional support by type of promotion including setting and costs, and new product development and global launch schedules.

As the market has changed, the secondary databases have mimicked those changes to include in-depth data on managed care, hospital treatment, global markets, etc. These data provided strategic support to marketers because they were actionable. They provided insight into *what* was happening in the marketplace and *why*. Like clues in a crime read by a good detective, they told a story of what happened and who did it. For example, a pharmaceutical marketer today could identify a problem–e.g., a major brand that has been deeply and quickly eroded by generics–and then identify the drivers of that event, e.g., substantial Medicaid business that immediately switched to generics. The databases are rich and detailed and provide multiple perspectives on the behavioral results that allow the marketer at least to infer cause. It is this actionability gained through the perspectives of all critical customers measured consistently over time that is also required in the next phase of the pharmaceutical industry's life.

## SECONDARY DATA REQUIREMENTS
## FOR THE NEXT MILLENNIUM

The features that make today's secondary resources so valuable must be replicated in the resources of the next industry phase. Specifically, all aspects of the market must be visible, and all future questions must be researchable.

### Data Must Represent All Market Segments

The value to the pharmaceutical industry of today's audit or secondary data is not only that it allows marketers to track all of the steps in the health care process (and therefore quantify market relationships and signal discontinuities) but also that it allows marketers to capture the drivers of those changes. Moreover, the capture of transactions and drivers must be complete and trendable, and the multiple data sources must be integratable, i.e., consistently measured. Only then can marketers interpret and act on a dynamic health care market. When the data have significant gaps–for example, when a market segment or transaction is not measured or is measured in units that are not coincident across all sources–the other available data diminish in value and usefulness, providing fewer and fewer pieces of the industry puzzle and potentially undermining the success of business planning and the effectiveness of strategic industry actions. The nature and size of the missing data, of course, makes a difference. If all of the market segments are effectively sampled, the planner can work effectively with the data remaining. But if the absent piece represents unique pieces of the market, as those pieces grow in size, their absence is more glaring and any conclusions that the marketer makes are less certain. For example, ten years ago when mail order represented an insignificant share of the retail business, it could be ignored, whereas today, knowledge of the dynamics of the mail-order channel is critical for successful marketing.

Currently, pharmaceutical marketers trying to get the most from secondary sources complain of the lack of detailed information about the hospital marketplace. We have purchases in a complete and trendable fashion, but the market drivers are frequently invisible. This failing is largely the result of multiple systems for and levels of data collection in individual hospitals which make it difficult to integrate data from one source with data from another. With the paucity of information on hospital decisions, critical information about individual therapies (e.g., cancer therapy, AIDS) is not provided in consistent, trendable secondary research resources. Hospitals, however, are just one example of an underrepresented customer segment. Data for clinics and home health care are also only partially captured. And the patient himself–a rapidly increasing *direct* customer of health care and medicine–is barely visible at all. In short, to be useful, the data of the next millennium must represent all customers of the new health care market.

### Data Measurements Must Address Future Concerns

To meet these value criteria, the collector and marketer of secondary data must understand the parameters (and the perimeters) of the market and its interconnections. The collector of longitudinal data must also avoid or limit measures that will be outdated in a few years time and would unnecessarily increase the size and decrease the manageability of the data. The supplier of health care "audit" data must gather all of those transactions that are anticipated to be critical in putting together the health care puzzle and gather them in a way that invites integrated analysis if actionable results are the desired outcome.

Secondary data collection and organization must also lend itself to frequent questioning and requestioning of the data. Research is an iterative process that makes working with secondary data something of a "Goldilocks and the Three Bears" exercise: one frequently has to try all three chairs to know which one is "just right." For the designer of secondary databases, that means that all possible levels or segmentations of the data–and all possible units of measurement–that the researcher *might* require for market interpretation and for solving business problems must be available in the database. A simple example should make the requirement clear. When many of today's secondary databases were developed, generics were minor factors in the market, if they existed at all. It would have been easy to classify products by brand and manufacturer rather than by molecule. Had that been done, however, the entire database would have had to be reclassified for investigation of today's pressing questions about generic impact on brand performance, etc. And although new data elements can sometimes be added at a later date, the longitudinal nature of the data and the visibility of specific trends is undermined by *ad hoc* changes.

## THE HEALTH CARE WORLD WE WILL LIVE IN

Incorporating questions and concerns of the future in database design is essential but difficult to do. This requirement is hard enough to meet when the market situation is stable. It is particularly daunting when the market is changing rapidly in multiple directions, and as yet unidentified market segments and market issues must be anticipated and incorporated into the data set.

Right now with the health care market in a state of considerable flux, many and varied future health care scenarios are possible. Consequently, many and varied data collection and distribution strategies are also possible. We at IMS have asked ourselves the questions: What will the markets of the future look like? Who will be the pharmaceutical purchase decision makers in the next century? What will distribution and use of health care entail? What databases, data elements–and data collection methods–will be needed to provide our clients with actionable information?

The answer to the last question depends on the answers to the first three, so we have hypothesized three distinct health care scenarios, each with its own secondary data requirements and each highlighting a major problem in data management and use that will have to be overcome no matter which of the future scenarios prevails. Specifically, Scenario #1 depicts the continuation of the current trend, i.e., the accelerated growth and eventual dominance of the health care system by for-profit managed care. This scenario, including the proliferation of data in tandem with managed care growth (plan data and formulary data, as well as physician data and pharmacy and other distribution channel data), spotlights the changing database user skills required to work with extensive microlevel data. Scenario #2 depicts the predominance of government-managed health care in U.S. medical delivery and coverage, including the development and desired use of 50 individual state databases. While suggesting exciting analytic opportunities, this scenario highlights the management and usage problems generated by multiple databases, each collecting different data sets; each formatted in unique ways; and each including distinct, unduplicated data elements. Scenario #3 anticipates a health care system divided between traditional health care and health care delivery methods (i.e., fee-for-service, managed care) and nontraditional, alternative therapies provided by nontraditional suppliers (e.g., acupuncturists, dance therapists, homeopaths) and distributed largely through currently unmonitored channels. This scenario offers great potential in evaluating new market opportunities, including copromotion and line extensions, but it also addresses the data collection and management problems of gathering information from unmonitored channels and integrating distinctly different data types to form a complete market picture.

### *Scenario #1: Expanded Managed Care Health Care*

The predominant view of most health care experts–and the major fear of most pharmaceutical manufacturers–is that managed care with restrictive formularies and intense pricing pressures will dominate health care delivery in the next century. Whether or not these expectations are realized, managed care and the issues of primary concern to managed care managers can no longer be excluded from critical industry research and planning. Managed care, therefore, will be central to all secondary research resources in the next millennium.

### *Overall Market Size and Characteristics*

Continued growth in HMO enrollment, particularly for–profit HMOs, that started in the late 1980s, could mean that by 2010 the total number of participants would grow to over 150 million–more than half of the U.S. population! In the 21st century, the most rapid growth in HMO enrollment is likely to be in plans that cover those eligible for Medicare. This growth would result both from younger HMO members staying with their plans when they become Medicare eligible and from carefully targeted marketing campaigns. This trend is likely to be encouraged by government, as it would provide one of the most effective ways of involving the private sector in containing escalating Medicare costs, enabling government to negotiate capitated fees with HMOs instead of fees for service with the providers.

Under this scenario, the most important provider response to the health care transformation is likely to be the growth of integrated health care organizations and of the more loosely affiliated preferred provider groups. Although still in existence, single practice physicians' offices and hospitals or clinics without group affiliations are likely to become more of a rarity, existing mainly in exceptional geographic or social environments.

## Managed Care Data Needs and Uses

The twofold response of the pharmaceutical companies to these developments is already being initiated in 1995. Companies are vastly increasing resources dedicated to managed care and provider network negotiations and establishing total disease management teams. Each of these developments creates vast new information needs, which–although they may have been anticipated, cannot be fully satisfied by the larger health care information companies (such as IMS) until early in the 21st century. This is due, in part, to the huge investment needed to create these databases, which often do not pay back until ten or so years from their inception; in part to the traditional concerns about data privacy and new parties needing to be educated about the long-term value of access to market research information; and also in part to the technological challenges, despite the ever-increasing power and decreasing costs of PCs and workstations.

## Managed Care Analyses Requirements and Tools

By 2010, most of the challenges to providing the newer databases and analytical tools are likely to have been overcome. The typical analyses that we anticipate being conducted under this scenario involve providers, plans, and the relationships between them and much more extensive patient disease management variables. The ability to carry out more in-depth analyses will be greatly facilitated by the explosion of client server architecture and the continuing decline in the cost of ever more powerful PC workstations.

*Visualization Techniques.* This technology will enable multiple access to complex data visualization tools, allowing managers at various levels to understand quickly the key information that affects their responsibilities and decision making. For example, pharmaceutical sales representatives would instantly be able to identify the plans or doctors in which their shares had deteriorated and could quickly revise their planning. Similarly, sophisticated data mapping tools such as Tactician™ and Conquest™ will enable district level managers to review their territory level deployment and to understand quickly the relative performance and competitive challenges within each of their territories. Increasingly, the data will be needed at the managed care plan level for action by national and regional accounts managers to prepare them for contract negotiations and for monitoring the extent to which there is compliance with and improved market share from the negotiated formulary status. In addition, we anticipate that data will be delivered electronically overnight from data providers to the database integrators, and, similarly, the data will be assimilated, quality assured, projected, and available to clients typically 24 to 48 hours later. Limitations related to timely provision of data will cease to be an issue. Instead, there will be increasing debate about how frequently it makes sense to review the data and revise action plans. By the year 2010, most of the pharmaceutical sales representatives will have grown up using what are now thought of as powerful PCs and will be expected to use sophisticated laptop software in their work routinely.

*Longitudinal Patient Databases.* Longitudinal patient databases that are currently in their infancy will still be growing by the year 2010 as the industry comes to appreciate the wealth of new applications of this data, particularly within a managed health care environment. Some of the applications already envisioned include monitoring disease progression, step therapy, improved estimates of overall disease incidence, comorbidity, and long-term side effect evaluation. In the future, this will be supplemented by more robust information on treatment effectiveness and outcomes measures taking into account, where appropriate, severity and risk adjustments. As the managed care organizations reach a near saturation level of enrollment, it is likely that they will start to focus to a greater extent on reducing treatment costs as their best opportunity to provide further profit growth. This is likely to lead to more sophisticated evaluations of preventive treatments, studies to evaluate earlier screening, and an even greater use of drugs such as cholesterol reducers and antihypertensives to reduce the long-term and expensive health care costs of heart disease (bypass surgery). Pharmaceutical companies will need access to patient databases both to justify to the managed care organizations earlier preventive interventions and to understand better the opportunity for new drug development.

*Integration of Claims Data and Practice Information.* Increasingly, analyses will be carried out at the managed care plan and doctor level to evaluate formulary compliance as well as the spillover from the plan and to estimate the accessible volume at the doctor level. Conceivably, by the year 2010, patient-level databases will begin to replace the current prescription and sales databases as the key information bases for compensation, planning, and sales force management. However, not showing whether the product was dispensed–a key drawback–means that most clients may continue to use either a prescription or sales tracking database for compensation. One of the biggest challenges for the patient-level databases will be to ensure that they cover treatment across channels, for example, at doctors' offices, hospitals, and clinics. It is currently not clear that this will be possible for large nationally representative samples, but the approaches that are likely to emerge would involve integrating claims and managed care databases with those of private practice providers and anonymously cross tracking the patient identities. There may be formidable challenges to produce these integrated patient databases, given the concerns about patient privacy. However, HCFA has already demonstrated with its Medicare databases that these can be produced while preserving anonymity.

## Marketing Research Uses of Managed Care Data

Imaginative uses of managed care data to direct marketing action exist today, most frequently in evaluating promotion response. Indeed, pharmaceutical clients are currently analyzing the impact of formulary restrictions on their brands to determine how aggressive their pricing must be to achieve their marketing objectives. Researchers use basic comparisons of prescription market share within tightly controlled and loosely controlled managed care formularies and national and/or total managed care markets to determine the level of formulary type impact on brand share. Additionally, researchers use promotion response techniques to evaluate the success of managed care pricing contracts in driving market share on a plan-by-plan basis.

In addition to evaluating the success of promotion, however, researchers today can also combine information about specific (e.g., hypertensive) disease severity and product share within different managed care settings to infer positioning of their own brand versus competitors' brands in treatment protocols. It is in this new zone combining treatment information with sales that we anticipate the greatest research uses in the next century. Marketing research of this type using large quantitative databases will be of value not only to managed care organizations for outcomes research but also to clinicians, who will be able to identify differential characteristics of patients who succeed on each therapy type.

## Scenario #2:
## State Government Dominated Managed Health Care

Although sweeping federal health care reform that guarantees universal access to basic health care is no longer a very likely scenario in the foreseeable future, the Clinton Administration has changed the face of the pharmaceutical industry forever. The push to control rapidly escalating health care costs has forced industry compliance with pricing guidelines. The days of high margins and easy profits have been replaced by a new national consciousness that demands accountability from all sectors of the health industry. The one common denominator of virtually all the competing health care reform plans is accountability.

## Characteristics of State-Regulated Managed Care

With the 1994 elections, however, health care is becoming a state, and not a federal, responsibility. State health insurance programs like Hawaii's and Oregon's have been scrutinized under a microscope by opposing parties in the national health care debate, and many states have spawned their own plans. New initiatives may include employer mandates for health insurance coverage, as in Hawaii, and the migration of Medicaid patients to HMOs, as in Oregon, Tennessee, Rhode Island, Kentucky, and Ohio. States will also have to set laws and policies that prevent skimming of low-risk patients by HMOs. Most forms of state health care reform involve partnerships between public and private health care planners and implementers. Employer mandates will require prioritization of services to manage costs. But, measuring the effectiveness of treatments and improving their effectiveness will be of great value regardless of who ultimately manages the provisioning of services. The information needs of both public and private parties are similar. Therefore, the demand for health care information services is easier to predict than the future political evolution of the health care industry.

## Information Needs of States: Regulated Managed Care

Proper service prioritization includes measuring the social costs of not providing services for basic health care. Claims data that include all diagnosis and treatment information for individual patients over long periods of time will be extremely valuable in improving cost-effective medical care. It will also make possible the identification of procedures and treatments that cost society more to *not* provide than to provide. This data is already at least partly available to some large HMOs but may be currently limited in time and scope. These databases will be huge, even by the standards of today's largest pharmaceutical databases.

Ultimately, the best data sources will be developed by companies with access to the information, experience in managing massive quantities of data, and the analytical forethought to anticipate the analyses that will be needed and the relative value of each piece of information that could or could not be carried. A whole new generation of analysis techniques will be needed to mine these massive data sources optimally. Hybrid techniques combining pattern recognition and artificial intelligence with heuristic searching algorithms will be developed. These techniques will leverage the visual aspects of human judgment that add the most value to the analysis process. Expert systems will automate the routine aspects of analysis that currently distract the attention and tax the limited memory of human analysts. Graphic user interfaces will require less effort for interaction, and visual information displays will be organized to provide rich cues for perceiving, storing, and retrieving information about causal relationships.

## Business Issues Requiring State Claims Databases

From the perspective of the providers of state-run managed care, the greatest value data analysis offers is the opportunity to increase the effectiveness and efficiency of health care delivery. However, because these are the needs of the purchasers of pharmaceuticals, pharmaceutical manufacturers, too, will focus their marketing attention on demonstrating that their products meet provider needs. Specifically, both customer and supplier will look to:

- Reducing the costs of pharmaceutical treatments
- Improving the cost-effectiveness of total health care solutions
- Evaluating patient population risk factors
- Prioritizing services offered for state reimbursement
- Evaluating service providers.

### Reducing the Costs of Pharmaceutical Treatments

To reduce the cost of therapies, payers (and providers) must be able to assess the costs of one therapy versus another balanced against treatment outcomes. Only then can the most cost-effective treatment be selected. With databases from different states, treatment costs will be accessible in different regions and different patient populations, guaranteeing that the best fit (i.e., the therapy that works for each individual patient type) will be selected first, with limited treatment trial and error.

To evaluate pharmaceutical treatment costs, researchers will track up to 3 million patients through the office record systems of 5,000 office-based physicians and merge that information with retail prescription transactions. This combination of resources will support evaluation of patient compliance, length of therapies (by product), and treatment outcomes at a state level. Although the outcomes information may be more sparse than preferred, it will still enable estimates to be made of the relative efficacy of alternative pharmaceutical therapies while guarding patient privacy.

## Improving the Cost-Effectiveness of Total Health Care Solutions

Large HMOs are currently developing and using databases linking total reimbursed treatments–both surgical and pharmaceutical–with patient outcomes to measure total health care costs. While today's data sources track hospital treatments as well as office treatments and prescriptions, they provide limited information about individual brands and pharmaceutical products that are not on their formularies. They may also suffer from limited outcomes information: claims records indicate when treatment is received but do not definitively indicate when a condition is cured.

To measure total therapy costs accurately in the next millennium, these databases will be supplemented with claims information from pharmaceutical benefits managers who process claims for many organizations with varied formulary policies. If, in addition, state government payers required state-insured patients to provide outcomes information on a regular basis, then this would provide a very powerful unbiased source of information for outcomes research. This information could also be fed back to practitioners to help the practitioners more effectively diagnose disease, prescribe treatments, implement treatments, and monitor the outcomes of interventions.

## Evaluating Patient Population Risk Factors

Although the United States' concerns with patient privacy have, until now, prevented the kind of encompassing population information available in Sweden, Germany, and France, new sources of patient data that mask individual patient identity can be a powerful source of estimating risks and, consequently, allocating resources for disease identification and treatment at a state level. Evaluating patient population risk factors is a logical extension of outcomes research. A large patient-level longitudinal database merged with individual patient demographics will provide a rich source for estimating the risks associated with providing services to specific patient demographic groups. We envision implementing these applications by linking geodemographic databases with hospital outcomes records. These databases provide a visual map of a geographic area along with detailed coding and visual representation of roads, power lines, sewers, manufacturing plants, and restaurants and population density distributions by demographic characteristics (all of which can be evaluated for health risks).

These databases, which contain a great deal of information from Census Bureau Tiger files, are new to the health care industry but have been used for many years by retail site location consulting firms. Their application to epidemiological research requires only the merger of hospital treatment records or, in the not-too-distant future, integration with patient-level medical histories tagged with the addresses of primary residences over time. Examples of the important actions that could be supported by these research tools are many. We will mention just one. Epidemiologists, for example, could determine if persons living near a nuclear power plant suffer from increased risks of cancer.

## Prioritizing Services Offered for State Reimbursement

Even the most liberal and humane of all state governments will not be able to provide reimbursement for all medical procedures. To evaluate which treatments should be reimbursed and which should not, systems for evaluating total treatment costs and estimating risk adjustments in patient populations will be integrated with systems that track patient care costs of untreated patients.

This system will be a challenge to build because it requires linking nontreatment events to subsequent events that cost the taxpayers money. We envision the necessary addition of financial data to patient data to make these judgments. Building these databases will require a great deal of judgment to limit the information collected and tracked to a manageable amount.

## Evaluating Service Providers

In the next century, managed care service providers will, necessarily, segment their service offerings, and they will look to secondary information to do so. Service quality is a subjective experience, but it is the key point of differentiation in most service industries. As Dr. Paul Ellwood and his Jackson Hole colleagues point out, comprehensive evaluation of service providers requires more than linking claims data with outcomes data to estimate the cost of producing physical outcomes. "Managed competition can only succeed if consumers select among competing health plans based on cost and quality" (1).

The principles of a customer-focused service orientation and effective service quality measurement are not unique to the medical industry. Experts in service quality measurement apply these principles across virtually every industry. The key to effective service quality measurement is to measure the subjective experiences of the service consumers as well as the objective parameters of service delivery. Perceived quality is a function of consumer values and expectations. Performance requirements change as competing providers demonstrate higher levels of service.

Taking our lead from other industries, we anticipate development of consumer-centered service quality audits as competition for managed care franchises heats up. These surveys, which will focus on consumer service expectations and requirements, will provide report cards for the major providers of managed care in the industry. But they will also serve to segment consumers by the aspects of service consumers value most highly. Finally, these surveys will track changing performance standards as expectations evolve over time with firsthand and vicarious experience.

### Scenario #3: Increased Impact of Alternative Therapies

In the still quasi-traditional world of 1995 health care, alternative medicine is a substantial but shadowy presence which is only infrequently reported to the patient's primary caregiver. Like over-the-counter medicines, alternative therapies could potentially increase in importance as health care system administrators look for lower cost alternatives to prescription pharmaceuticals, surgical procedures, and expensive technological advances and as patients look to cheaper and more customized care. While data are gathered on OTC medicines, there is currently no monitoring of sales, patient visits, concomitant therapies, and provider numbers or characteristics in nontraditional therapies. Alternative medicines are an increasing force in health care whose strength and role has been unmeasured to date.

### Overall Market Size and Characteristics

Five years ago, in a kinder and gentler health care system, more than one-third of the American population used alternative or unconventional therapies, according to David Eisenberg's 1992 study (2). The type of therapy included in Eisenberg's study ranged from dietary regimens to acupuncture and massage therapy. The conditions for which these therapies were used included a variety of chronic problems (backache, gastrointestinal problems, headache, cancer). Projecting his survey results on a national basis, Eisenberg estimated that "the number of ambulatory visits to providers of unconventional therapy in 1990 was 425 million [representing 61 million people, which] exceeds the estimated 388 million visits in 1990 to all primary care physicians (general and family practitioners, pediatricians and specialists in internal medicine) combined." Eisenberg further estimates that $14 billion was spent on unconventional therapy in 1990 in the U.S., which "is comparable to the out-of-pocket expenditure for all hospital care in the United States in 1990 ($12.8 billion) and it is nearly half the amount spent out of pocket for all physicians' services in the United States." In addition, (not surprisingly), the cost of alternative medicine treatments is lower, on average, than that of traditional medicine, with the mean charge per visit to a provider being $27.60 in 1990 (2). When coupled with the reimbursement information, the level of total expenditure is even more impressive. Fifty-five percent of alternative therapies were unreimbursed by a third party payer. Of the remaining 45% that was at least partially reimbursed, one-third was totally reimbursed and two-thirds was only partially covered by a third-party payer.

Recent action by the NIH underscores the increasing importance of this virtually opaque market segment. Alternative medicine is now a recognized focus of the National Institutes of Health, and there are currently 42 research grants (totaling $1.2 million) nationally, testing the efficacy of such treatments as music therapy, dance therapy, Qi gong, bee pollen treatments, and acupuncture. Six fields of therapy are included under the general rubric of alternative medicine: nutrition and lifestyle regimens; mind and body control; ethnic medicine, yoga, homeopathy, and acupuncture; structural manipulation; bioelectrical applications; and pharmacological treatments.

The most important aspect of this direction in U.S. health care, however, is that it heralds the emergence of the strongest health care and pharmaceutical customer, the patient.

*Alternative Therapies Driven Data Needs*

Let us assume that patients increasingly turn to these alternatives because they provide the critical caring and interactive components of treatment that are increasingly absent in a hurried, time restricted managed care environment and because they are substantially less expensive than other health care alternatives. Should this happen (as, indeed, it is already happening) there are critical factors about the use of alternative therapies that a collector and analyst of secondary data must address:

- The use of unconventional medicine is widespread now and growing, and there is no available benchmark.

- It generates substantial numbers of patient visits and dollars and is a potential source of additional profit growth to the industry.
- It is generally un- or underreported to the conventional medical practitioner, and its impacts on outcomes are unknown.
- Less than half of the payments for alternative therapies are reimbursed by a third-party payer, so claims data cannot supply the missing information.

How will marketers and new product developers know the level, the concomitant use, and the competitive market set that includes these therapies when these therapies have such radically different–and currently un-audited–distribution channels? How will they know what is important to the patient's health care decisions without this information? It is clear that in *this* brave new world, secondary information on the distribution, use, pricing, practitioner, and patient profiles of alternative therapies *must* be collected, organized, and analyzed for health care marketing to be as fact based as it is today. What might be available? What business issues could be addressed? How might it be collected? Who would use it? How would it be used?

Business Issues Requiring Alternative Therapy Data

*Market Opportunity Assessment.* The description of the market is often the first requirement of a marketer. Indeed, the very first question, "Should I bother with this area?" can only be answered with an accurate market size and competitive set definition. Once the market configuration and value are assessed, however, marketers need to understand where and how much the market overlaps with more traditional areas. Only then, of course, can they determine opportunities for joint ventures, copromotions, and licensing and acquisition deals and ascertain reasons to protect against possible switching away from their own products.

*Identification of Patient Customer Needs.* As discussed above, the growth of alternative therapies signals the increased market strength of the patient. Historically, the patient was presumed to have little say in his own therapeutic decisions. In fact, when certain physician specialties were deciding on treatment, patient preference exerted a *negative* effect on treatment choice. However, increased competition among health care providers, together with new sensitivity to interpatient biological differences, means that already today (and with certainty in the future) the patient can and will assert authority in selection of provider and therapy. The result will be the critical need of the pharmaceutical industry to understand patient needs and choice behavior and the ways to influence them.

*Pharmaceutical Resource Allocation.* The growth in new customers, combined with pressures to reduce manufacturer costs, means that the pharmaceutical industry must be particularly careful in deploying resources. To a certain extent, the pattern of the present day is "find a new customer, reduce promotion to the older one." This is evident in the tidal wave industry movement to pharmaceutical benefits management and managed care and away from traditional physician detailing. Ironically, this all-or-nothing pattern is similar to the move away from detailing in the pharmacy ten years ago, when the pharmaceutical industry went from direct distribution to wholesaler distribution. Pharmaceutical manufacturers of the next millennium, however, cannot afford to neglect *any* of their customers. They will need them all. Alternative therapies information will offer an opportunity to assess the purchase power of patient groups in individual therapy areas and to deploy the appropriate level of promotional resources to each market segment according to its potential return.

*Outcomes Research and Cost-Effectiveness Studies.* From the perspectives of the pharmaceutical industry manufacturers and managed care providers, therapies must prove their worth in dollars and cents. Alternative therapies hold the key to accurate assessment of that worth, either as monotherapy or as combination therapy–synergistic or detrimental. In fact, the present-day absence of alternative therapies from patient records and physician knowledge indicates that today's outcomes research and cost-effectiveness studies are potentially flawed and may be inadequate for some decision support applications. Only when *all* therapies that the patient takes have been accounted for can comparisons of effectiveness and better return on the health care dollar be made. A corollary consideration, too, is that Phase IV studies (or postmarketing surveillance), which are increasingly the norm, must be able to identify contraindicated medicines and procedures and so patients and providers may be advised accordingly.

## Data Availability and Collection Methods

Key to monitoring of alternative therapies is collection of data at the point of purchase, at the user level, and at the payer level. Alternative therapies are like over-the-counter medicines in that the provider of care–and the ultimate decision maker about whether and when care should be given–is the consumer/patient. Surprisingly, today's pharmaceutical manufacturers often spend more planning time (and certainly more worrying time) trying to understand patient compliance issues (i.e., whether and why the patient follows the physician's directions) than they do trying to understand patient self-care behaviors. The new importance of alternative therapies requires full and ongoing collection of information from the patient about his or her health care behaviors and the motivations for those behaviors. We envision data collection at the patient level provided by very large household panels (a kind of hybrid to the household panels of today's consumer market and the government-sponsored National Health Surveys) supplying detailed information about all treatments, including alternative therapies and OTC products. The households, of course, will be sampled to represent all market segments. Coincidentally, purchases at health food stores and other channels of alternative care distribution will be audited, as will dispensing providers. Additional information based on insurance claims data must also be gathered and codified. Data suppliers will face the daunting task of integrating these data sources to get the 360 degree perspective that will be needed. This effort will be difficult and will require database nesting. Undoubtedly, the effort will drive database suppliers to consolidate and merge, much as their pharmaceutical customers and others in the health care industry have consolidated. But this process, in fact, replicates the original innovative collection and database development efforts of the 1960s that produced the rich audit system of today's pharmaceutical industry. And it will, again, encourage innovative marketing research uses.

Marketing Research Uses of Alternative Therapy Databases

The availability of ongoing information about choices made by all of the pharmaceutical industry's customers will put marketing researchers in the catbird seat. Consumer-based industries have always depended heavily on marketing research because it offered one of the few ways that marketers could understand and segment the needs of their large and diffuse market and then tailor their products and promotions to meet those needs. Theirs was a highly competitive market, and the constant fight for market share required frequent market readings. The pharmaceutical industry, by contrast, had well-defined customer segments that companies knew in a personal way through their nationwide sales forces. And, unlike the consumer market, there was relatively little they could do to create–or inhibit–"usage occasions." Their marketing attention was directed at monitoring their growth and competitive strength. The health care market of the next millennium will be a blend of the pharmaceutical market of the past with added components of business to business and a strong consumer market. Research must be able to address these multiple and complex needs. Examples of the kind of research that will be done might be complex promotion response studies, integration of consumer and distribution data using geographic mapping techniques, and variants of patient record studies.

*Promotion Response Studies.* Today promotion response studies in the health care market usually look at marketing mix for one product only, and, for the purposes of assessment, assume the product's promotional intervention alone differentiates the test group from the control. The impact of competitors' counterpromotions are generally ignored because large sample audits on competitive activity are not available. These analyses provide good estimates of promotional impact in the context of current competitive activity because that activity is equally distributed across test and control groups. These analyses do not allow the product manager to understand the positive and negative synergistic effects that his promotional programs will have conditional upon varying levels of competitor promotions. In the world of the future, however, multiple coincidental promotional efforts can be assessed simultaneously by combining point-of-purchase promotion and deal evaluations with specific consumer promotions (e.g., television advertising) for all products competing in a market. The advantage of this type of modeling is that it allows the simulation of conditional strategies that will lead to optimal allocation of marketing resources. Using these techniques, marketers will have a better understanding of their product's brand equity, and because patterns of asymmetrical cross elasticities between competitors will clearly define the dominant players, marketers will be able to avoid self-destructive marketing wars.

*A 360 Degree Regional Market Perspective.* In an ongoing effort to get closer to the customer, many pharmaceutical manufacturers have instituted (or reinstituted) regional business units. These field-based offices are currently able to assess their own competitive efforts and success as distinct from the performance of the company as a whole and by comparison to the performance of other company regional business units. The goal is immediate and specific course correction, if needed, rather than today's reliance on the home office to react to the buildup of warning signals from the field before changing direction. The availability of prescriber, plan, and promotion activity establishes a sense of cause and effect now at the district level. With the integration of alternative therapy (including OTC drug) information, regional managers will understand their business environment enough to *anticipate* market changes.

*Patient-Based Treatment of Diseases.* With a variant on the currently used patient record studies, in which health care providers keep patient diaries that enable researchers to capture implicit determinants of product selection, marketing researchers will be able to support the strategic and tactical needs of new clients. Specifically, in the next millennium, with patients keeping "care" diaries, researchers will be able to capture patients' motivations for selection of providers and treatment modalities. Analysis of this information will provide critical direction to government agencies, managed care, and hospitals in planning provision of services.

## SUMMARY AND CONCLUSIONS

Not surprisingly, exploration of a variety of alternative health care future scenarios suggests an expansion of our research resources in the next millennium will be necessary to capture the needs of multiple customers (many of them new) and the increased diversity in health care delivery. Moreover, we anticipate that customers on both sides of the aisle will demand information to support their own decision making. For example, in our various scenarios, we have hypothesized patients selecting managed care plans, patients selecting therapy types, managed care plans selecting treatment protocols, physicians and epidemiologists matching therapies with patients, state governments allocating treatment resources, and more. All of these are in addition to today's selection of pharmaceutical products by physicians and managed care organizations. Across all scenarios, in fact, we anticipate increases in available information, additional tools to access and use that information, and increased marketing capabilities.

### New Information for the Next Millennium

In keeping with the obvious ascendancy of the customer in health care decision making, the centerpiece of new information resources will be longitudinal patient-level information. Most critical–and innovative–will be the integration of providers, plan variables, and patient disease management variables for delineation of their interrelationships. Use of health care across all channels (including currently unaudited channels) at state and regional levels will be enhanced for integration with the patient databases. Further embellishment will come from newly included financial and environmental variables to map exactly the patient, the treatment, and the costs of health care. Given the complexity of the information needed, we anticipate a blend of transaction audits and survey methodologies to collect the data.

### New Tools for Information Presentation and Analysis

The magnitude of available data by itself could lead to technological suffocation and the extinction of sensitive analyses (i.e., so much data, there is no time to think). Happily, however, we see new tools to help analysts quickly understand and act on the information at hand. Specifically, visualization and mapping tools will speed interpretation of information for business and medical uses. The delivery of the data, of course, will be even quicker than it is today, with 24-48 hour turnaround made possible by improvements in client server architecture.

## New Marketing and Therapeutic Decision Capabilities

The availability of microlevel information in almost, if not exact, real time will enable the marketer to review his or her market performance on a daily basis. The pressing question, therefore, will be what frequency best supports marketing actions. This is not a question for information suppliers, of course, whose objective is to satisfy all users' needs; however, we imagine that rather than daily reforecasts, marketers will finally be able to follow the suggestion of business pundits like Russell Ackhoff, who advise daily review of forecast assumptions.

Complete information will also enable monitoring and tracking of compliance at many critical levels. These levels include plan monitoring for volume-based contract fulfillment, patient compliance monitoring, and long-term cost-effectiveness/outcomes monitoring which will provide marketers with the opportunity to adjust tactics and–when necessary–strategies. Monitoring and tracking capabilities will also enable improved health care delivery.

Finally, rich data resources provided with speed and analytic tools will enhance marketers', managers', and government's abilities to allocate resources (both promotional and therapeutic) appropriately and, in general, to manage their businesses on a level that clearly defines the forest while detailing all of the trees.

The brave new world of information–particularly secondary resources– that we envision in the next millennium, therefore, does not have a different shape from today's data resources. But it does have many colors that today's information does not. Used well, these new resources will support better targeting and niche marketing and overall less wasteful marketing. Our optimistic conclusion, consequently, is that even if the maturing U.S. health care industry of the next millennium generates lower revenues than it did in the 1980s, use of information resources will make it more profitable and robust than it was in its carefree youth.

## REFERENCES

1. Lansky, Knudsen, Wetzler. Outcomes accountability. April 1993. Discussion draft.

2. Eisenberg, et al. Unconventional medicine in the United States. N Engl J Med 1993;328:246-52.

# A Pharmaceutical Marketing Plan for the 21st Century: Primary Research Prospects

Robert N. Zelnio
Deborah K. Bertram

## *INTRODUCTION*

Marketing research is no stranger to change. As a corporate staff function, it has been restructured, reorganized, expanded, downsized, globalized, regionalized, etc., for the past 20 years or so. Why should we be concerned with such an old and worn-out topic now? Because the changes that have occurred during the last five years have been and those likely to occur during the next five years will be unprecedented and fundamental, affecting what questions are asked, who is asking them, how and by whom they are answered, and the types of actions to which they lead. These changes will be driven by the external economic and political forces that are reshaping the total health care environment rather than by the whims and politics of internal management.

Pressure on pricing and controlling costs is the overriding theme shaping the context in which all other changes will occur. This is the information age, and more than ever before, competitive advantage and ultimate success will be determined by the access to and application of information

Robert N. Zelnio, Ph.D., is President of Paragon Research & Consulting, Paoli Executive Green II, Suite 301, 43 Leopard Road, Paoli, PA 19301-1517. Deborah K. Bertram, M.B.A., is President of Bertram Group Consulting, Lee's Summit, MO.

[Haworth co-indexing entry note]: "A Pharmaceutical Marketing Plan for the 21st Century: Primary Research Prospects." Zelnio, Robert N., and Deborah K. Bertram. Co-published simultaneously in *Journal of Pharmaceutical Marketing & Management* (Pharmaceutical Products Press, an imprint of The Haworth Press, Inc.) Vol. 10, No. 2/3, 1996, pp. 61-107; and: *Pharmaceutical Marketing in the 21st Century* (ed: Mickey C. Smith) Pharmaceutical Products Press, an imprint of The Haworth Press, Inc., 1996, pp. 61-107. Single or multiple copies of this article are available from The Haworth Document Delivery Service [1-800-342-9678, 9:00 a.m. - 5:00 p.m. (EST)].

success will be determined by the access to and application of information for strategic decision making. It is past time for marketing research to step up and take advantage of the opportunities presented. As a discipline, marketing research must evolve to a new level that truly meets the needs of pharmaceutical companies. In any company where such strategic changes are ignored or resisted, the primary marketing research function will not survive. It will be outsourced, and secondary data management will be the only internal remnant of the traditional marketing research function.

In 1993, it was concluded, based on a qualitative study, that the needs of upper management were unmet by the services provided by marketing research. This report called for three paradigm shifts: a need to focus on the future, a need to form partnerships with marketing, and a need to enhance the professional stature of marketing research (1). According to a follow-up quantitative study in 1994, there has been progress toward better partnerships. However, there has been little progress in enhancing marketing research's professional stature, and more important, upper management remains skeptical about the contribution marketing research makes to planning for the future. More firmly put, this study reports that "senior management remains unimpressed not only with marketing researchers' marketplace sophistication but even with the level of their technical job skills" (2). Another observer, in commenting upon some of marketing research's shortcomings, has concluded that "a somewhat different marketing research philosophy is needed in order to succeed" (3). He calls for a shift from quality control research to the more proactive quality improvement research. This research builds upon these efforts by seeking to:

1. Identify the factors that will influence primary pharmaceutical marketing research in the next 5 years
2. Predict how these factors will affect primary pharmaceutical marketing research
3. Offer conclusions on how marketing research, as a discipline, might respond to these factors.


## METHODS

The data on which this analysis is based were gathered by six individual depth interviews and three group depth interviews with pharmaceutical marketing research executives. All interviews were conducted during the period from late February through March of 1995. In all, 15 individuals were interviewed.[1]

## RESULTS AND DISCUSSION

Reported in this section are the factors that respondents indicate have shaped and will continue to shape the nature of pharmaceutical marketing and marketing research. As such, they will also have implications for primary marketing research services. The information in this section will also offer to explain the impact of these factors.

### Demand for Marketing Research Services Is on the Rise

There is general agreement that the demand for marketing research services has increased and will continue to increase. The increasing reliance of internal clients on marketing research's services is highly evident. It is a consistent theme that almost no decisions are made without marketing research.

> *I think more and more all important decisions that are made now are research based. So I think that's changed the objectives because people aren't going ahead and doing big programs or making big decisions unless they have some good, solid facts behind why they've made those decisions.*

There is some disagreement, however, on the form of the services that will be demanded and the sources of supply that will be used to meet demand. These issues aside, the view that the demand for marketing research will continue to increase has been fueled by a number of factors.

First, respondents claim that the perceived value of marketing research services has increased. Several hypotheses can be offered for this increase. The PMRG, for example, has devoted much effort to the technical training of researchers and to programs aimed at increasing the professionalism and visibility of marketing research departments. Similarly, proactivity has been a consistent issue of discussion within the PMRG. Another hypothesis is that the practice of rotating personnel through marketing research as part of the developmental process may contribute to an increase in perceived value. Odd as it may seem, this practice, which is normally blamed for the devaluation of marketing research, could have exposed future upper managers to the potential richness of marketing research services. It is conceivable that all of the processes suggested by these hypotheses have collaborated to enhance the perceptions of marketing research.

*All I can tell you is that the need for information and the value of information placed on it by current management is a lot higher than it was by former management. So we have marketing research basically on the executive committee instead of someplace down somewhere reporting to marketing.*

Second, the increase in demand undoubtedly stems from the fact that marketing successes come harder in the present market. Gone are the days when even me-too drugs can be marketed profitably. And, with increasing external pressures on pharmaceutical marketing and product development, mistakes are more costly. So, it is not surprising that no decisions are made without the benefit of marketing research.

A third potential factor is the increase in the number of marketing research's internal clients. In the past, marketing research almost solely serviced product management's needs, but now more product development, clinical study, and business decisions are relying on marketing research, as is further discussed below.

A fourth factor will have more impact in the future. As the nature of pharmaceutical products changes, it is hypothesized that the structure and functioning of the market for these products will change. Genetic engineering and recombinant products are expected to alter the delivery of and market for pharmaceuticals. As a result, it is expected that the demand for marketing research services will increase along with the increased need to understand and capitalize on these marketplace changes.

*As we start to see products or potential products arising out of our alliances on gene technology and the like, I can't believe the market for those products will operate in the standard way that we currently see. My hypothesis, therefore, is that the demands for research will be different, but I just can't see what they are.*

### Marketing Research Technology Has Outpaced Its Application

The technology of marketing research has advanced faster than the ability to capitalize on it. Significant advances have been made as a result of the increased capabilities of personal computers and more knowledgeable computer users. The volume of data that can be accessed is enormous. Data that did not exist or was beyond the user's reach is now available. The speed with which data can be accessed, processed, and presented has increased dramatically. Complex research techniques that previously required main frame capabilities and therefore resided within academic institutions or with a minority of "elite" researchers have enjoyed more widespread use and distribution. Furthermore, the explosion of communications technology has opened up new research approaches.

> *I think we're doing things differently now. I think we're doing computer-assisted telephone interviews. We're doing videodepth interviews, teledepth interviews a lot more than we used to in order to cut down on travel time. I think we're using technology to shave time and expense wherever possible.*

But pharmaceutical marketing researchers share the world-at-large's love-hate relationship with technological advancement. While technology may have increased access to many needed tools, the disadvantages of increasing technology are all too obvious. Just as audio entertainment equipment has advanced to the point where it can produce sound quality that humans cannot appreciate, technology has advanced beyond our capabilities to use it fully. Using advanced statistical techniques, marketing researchers can build ever more complex market models, involving more products and product lines, more features/benefits, and more ability to cope with market uncertainty such as product entry/egress. This ability has tended to foster an unnecessarily complex view of the market which is reflected in the models being constructed.

> *I see the quantitative models expanding exponentially in the number of people that you have to bring into the model to get an understanding of what's going to be the product acceptance and how is that based on price and other things.*

At least for the present, humans are still making the decisions in the marketplace and, in making these decisions, they do not process (and, indeed, could not process) all of the information that researchers can include in models. Consistent with this finding is the observation that respondents are increasingly unable to complete the questionnaires designed to gather the data required for parameterization of these complex models. Thus, the models must be simplified to reflect more accurately the nature of the decision-making processes.

While we have increased our technological/methodological capabilities, the models presently employed do not meet all of marketing research's clients' needs. As will be discussed, this has led to the demand for new methods–both qualitative and quantitative. Respondents predict that they will, eventually, make even greater use of the new technologies at our disposal. They predict the increasing provision of questionnaires by floppy disk and by downloading via modem and on-line service. But they add that more computer survey methods leading to the increased proportion of computer literate respondents in our samples will lead to biased results. And, while there will be more research tools available, communicating the results to management will tax marketing research's written and verbal skills.

### Information Overload Is Overwhelming

There can be no denial that the amount of data available to the pharmaceutical industry about customers, products, competitors, and issues is growing exponentially. This has always been a relatively information-rich industry, and now technology is facilitating the proliferation of data and databases. Whereas audit information has historically dealt with aggregated market statistics, information is now provided at the individual physician level. Moreover, information has been expanded in keeping with pharmaceutical marketing's expanding customer base.

> *These databases today can count the prescriptions not only by physician and product, but by physician and product and type of plan and specific type of plan. You didn't have data for it before, and you couldn't do it reliably before.*

> *The proliferation of data and databases that we didn't have before is changing. For example, any of the companies that have PBMs as part of their business now have access to a whole spectrum of data that wasn't available before.*

For the most part, this added information has been databased incrementally, without displacing previously available audit data. So, not only is there now added information on new market segments, but also this information and the data on previously existing segments is provided at successively more detailed levels. The sheer volume and detail of this information along with its availability on-line or in locally accessible databases is nothing short of overwhelming. One respondent's admission that *"[s]ome data will never be used"* is typical among these marketing researchers. As with basic marketing research technology, the human and corporate capacity to use all of this data has not kept up with the amount and level of data available.

What is more, this trend will continue with the ongoing development and release of new databases and reports. At some point, though, company funding for incremental resources will run out. Those resources that have not maintained their relevancy to current market issues will be discontinued. Syndicated studies may not always be widely purchased because the information needs of companies having specific service agreements with their customers could be very different. Difficult choices will have to be made among the remaining options, unless significant price reductions are implemented by the developers and providers. But even price reductions may not be enough, as eventually customers for this information can be expected to purchase only what they can use.

The proliferation of databased audit information and syndicated studies, however, may be just the tip of the iceberg. On-line services such as the Internet, the World Wide Web, and the commercial on-line services provide access to literally unlimited quantities of published information. Furthermore, the interactive networks available on-line already provide spontaneous access to qualitative data in the form of messages in patient and professional user groups or forums. In the future, these services may provide the means to obtain audit and/or survey data directly from physicians' offices on a daily basis. The appeal of real-time data and information access as a means to understanding the rapidly changing environment will lead to even greater use of on-line services.

At present, however, effective application of discrete databases and on-line information is limited. The volume and organization of information available place much of it beyond the grasp of end users. They do not yet have the mechanisms in place for routine, broad-based, systematic searches. For example, those who use the commercial services or have begun to "surf the net" generally have identified only a few good sources, forums, or user groups on which to rely. And end-users are not equipped to summarize the information obtained from databases and on-line services. Software development is needed to enable data integration and simultaneous queries of multiple databases to establish crucial data links. These are powerful capabilities which can produce significant advantages for the companies who harness them.

Thus, more than ever before, the specific information accessed and, indeed, the volume of information marketers are able to use may provide a competitive edge. Access, however, may not remain as open as is presently the case. Through pharmaceutical company ownership of pharmaceutical benefits management companies (PBMs) and other vertically and horizontally integrated entities, some databases have become proprietary. Such ownership may lead to the beginning of a new era marked by differential access to data that is dependent on factors other than willingness and ability to pay. Prior to this divergence, companies had equal access, and access in and of itself did not provide a competitive edge. In the future, the ultimate determination of the advantage derived from data access, however, will remain in the hands of those responsible for analyzing and applying information to marketing strategy.

> *If I'm Merck, I don't know that I'm real anxious to give the rest of the pharmaceutical industry every bit of information out of Medco.*

By answering in great detail the question of *what* is going on in the marketplace, the plethora of secondary data will continue to redefine the need for traditional primary research. More primary research dollars will be used to understand *why* something is happening, to predict future market movement, and to develop and evaluate potential value-added programs and services. The availability of prescriber- and patient-level data also allows easier identification of specific subsets of customers for recruitment to participate in primary research. And even the most interactive databases contain historical data, reporting what has already happened. Models that integrate secondary data with primary research results to develop predictive scenarios of the future will provide real value.

### Multiple Decision Makers Lead to New Marketing Audiences

The single most discussed factor by these respondents is the number of different audiences who must be addressed by primary research. Long gone are the days of the physician as the sole research target. The decision-making process for the use of pharmaceutical products has become very complex within an environment of cost control and managed care.

> *The audience that we deal with is changing. It's becoming a much more complex effort to make sure that all of the stakeholders in the decision-making process on whether the drug is going to be utilized or not are addressed.*

> *The buyers of our products and the buyers of health care are changing. So, therefore, where before if we could influence the physician and he could and would write our product, that was the end of the game. But now, you can have every one of your physicians believing that you have the best product, but if it's not available on the closed formulary they belong to, then you don't get any business.*

The stakeholders in this process are multiple and varied, and the anticipated trend is toward even more complexity. Respondents predict that research with physicians will continue to be a relevant part of the mix, as long as physicians' decision-making authority is not totally constrained by the majority of formularies. However, the motivations of everyone involved in the decision process will also have to be understood and factored into marketing strategies. In addition to physicians, the variety of groups involved in the decisions about pharmaceutical care include:

- Pharmacists, Pharm.D.s, and pharmacy directors
- Pharmaceutical benefits managers
- Group purchasing organizations
- Managed care administrators
- Fee-for-service insurers
- Employers
- Physician assistants
- Nurses, nurse practitioners, and midwives
- Patients.

The greatest challenge over the next few years will be to identify accurately the decision makers in any given situation. Although the groups listed above can and will be targeted, they play different roles in each organization or system at different points in time. And, in many cases, the individuals with the specific responsibilities of interest to marketing research from one organization to the next may have entirely different positions and titles, not to mention educational and experiential backgrounds. This situation may preclude research designs based on uniformly questioning a sample from any of the above categories. It also adds another step to the research process: the identification of the correct decision maker/respondent in each individual organization.

To make matters worse, the populations of decision makers in some of these groups are very small, meaning that the efforts of pharmaceutical marketers will have to become even more targeted to focus on fewer individuals across a broader array of categories. Interactions among the decision makers will also need to be discerned by marketers so they can work in concert with multiple audiences. Profiling, rather than sampling, will provide the most actionable information. Other specialized groups within pharmaceutical companies will have better and more direct access to this type of information than marketing research will.

Thus, the complexity of the decision-making process is compounded by the need to map each decision chain separately and repeatedly as structural changes resulting from mergers/acquisitions and other forms of evolution occur. Additional decision-maker categories may develop as the result of ongoing health care reform and restructuring.

*As far as marketing research, I think it's become more difficult to understand the decision process because there are many more decision-makers. So instead of talking to one or two people on the medical side, now you're talking to four or five or six people who are overseeing the use of drugs in the managed care or in the hospital plus the people who are actually making decisions to use the drug.*

### Patients Will Be the Driving Force of Health Care

The emerging influence of patients among the multiple audiences to be targeted is particularly noteworthy. Traditionally, patients were left out of the decision-making process and simply told by physicians what medications were prescribed and how to take them. In response to a variety of phenomena, all of that has changed dramatically. First, it is logical that, as the ultimate end users of prescription products, patients' decision-making power will continue to increase. Facilitating their claim to meaningful decision-making participation is the fact that today's general population is better educated and has access to more medical information than previous generations.

Second, the recognition of these facts has, in the past few years, caused patients to become the targets of prescription pharmaceutical marketing with the increase in direct-to-consumer campaigns. Thus, assisted by industry-sponsored educational programs and direct-to-consumer advertising, patients are becoming more knowledgeable about health issues, disease states, and treatments. The industry itself is preparing patients for a more meaningful decision-making role. Respondents predict that patients' appetites for medical information will continue to expand and drive trends such as self-medication and exploration and use of various alternative therapies such as acupuncture, herbal medicine, and Rolfing®.

*There's also an increasing role of consumers in deciding about their health care these days. They're much more educated and knowledgeable.*

A third trend contributing to the growing importance of the patient in pharmaceutical marketing and, hence, marketing research is the increase in Rx-to-OTC switching. This is not only consistent with patients' increased decision-making roles but is also fueled by the government's and managed care's motivation for cost reduction. Pushing Rx products to the other side of the counter should introduce competitively lowered costs. In any event, it tends to convert products from reimbursable to nonreimbursable. For their part, pharmaceutical companies often see a product switch to OTC as an antigeneric strategy. This may be why some respondents suggest that the industry adopt the mission of shifting power to patients.

*I personally believe one of the long-term approaches of the industry is to bring about that sort of effect. To have patient demand. I don't believe we'll see it as a significant force in the industry within the next five years, but long-term, I think we must work toward that.*

Fourth, respondents predict that the higher and higher out-of-pocket fees patients will be required to pay for their medications will result in more involved patients. The shifts to OTC, of course, are consistent with this prediction. But, in addition, insurers and employers are expected to change the mix of reimbursement, increasingly shifting the burden to patients. In part, this will happen because of the power employers have to dictate medical insurance benefits to their employees. It will also happen, however, as formularies become more and more closed and as more restrictions are placed on prescribing, such as preauthorization and/or specified prescribing priorities. These phenomena mean that patients will be faced with increased copayments and more total self-pay for off-formulary prescribing.

*I think long-term we will see it because I think people are going to be forced to pay for more and more things out of their own pocket. I think they're going to want to be better educated about what they're getting, and I think they're going to speak up.*

*I think General Motors is going to make the decision that the whole corporation is going to get a specific kind of health care. The patient is going to have very little to say about that. I think what will happen is, economically, General Motors will be passing the burden. I think issues of copay if you want to go outside of the formulary, etc.–they will be passing that on to the patients.*

Marketing researchers are just beginning to explore the numerous factors that must be understood to do studies at the patient level. Among these are the need to know how to reach and talk to patients; recognition of the impact of lifestyle, family context, and psychological issues on patient-generated demand; and the need to affect compliance as well as product requests of physicians. Massive amounts of primary marketing research with the patient/consumer will be required to assure the successful targeting of patients. Furthermore, the development of patient databases has yet to emerge.

*We're entering into a new therapeutic area. We know that there's a patient component to therapy. So we're more likely to go right to the patients as well as to physicians to try and understand that dimension, especially if there's an emotional component involved.*

*Patient data will be the replacement of prescriptions, eventually. It will be used to judge business and calculate compensation, once technology improves on administrative databases.*

### Market Targeting Operationalizes the Focus on New Audiences

Pharmaceutical representatives have traditionally profiled the physicians, pharmacists, and hospitals in their territories. But this information was usually not available at the levels of the organization responsible for crafting marketing strategies. Not until the advent of call reporting systems and individual physician level databases has it been possible for pharmaceutical marketers to practice market segmentation as it was conceived in the 1950s. The most recent databases developed have made and will continue to make such targeted programs easier, if not feasible, to implement and evaluate. Both customer profiles and geographic areas will be used to develop the targeting matrix. Consistent with the theory of segmentation, pharmaceutical marketers implementing such targeting should become better at meeting the needs of their customers. This, of course, should lead to greater success in the marketplace.

Product management is presently targeting customers individually, although it is still inefficient to prepare individual-level promotional materials.

*The products that we deal with are very targeted products, and we're actually looking, in the case of a couple of our products, at profiling every single physician that we target. Not just in terms of their prescribing habits per se, but in terms of how many patients do they see, what type of practice do they have, and what sort of affiliations do they have. But it is going down to the physician level.*

As a result, marketing research now has added responsibilities for conducting research in ways consistent with target marketing. Marketing research must understand, maintain, and use the databases crucial to target marketing. Samples must be drawn from the target segments. Survey research must collect the data needed to classify respondents into target segments correctly. Individual physician prescribing data available from databases should be correlated with the survey research data on a segment-by-segment basis to model the behavior of target segments more validly.

*Even in the general research with physicians and the like, it's much more specific populations. The organization is targeting more specifically so, therefore, the research ought to as well.*

Interestingly, the increased implementation of segmentation strategies is proving to be a recursive process. The more involved product managers become with target marketing, the more they learn to refine their targeting. So marketing research must be flexible, aiming primary research at a moving definition of products' targets.

*I think one of the changes that's starting and will continue is defining who the customers are. I think we will have a much clearer picture of who the key customers are that we're going after. We will be going less and less after broad specialty classifications and more and more targeting in on specific kinds of physicians within specialties. Probably the same will be true of managed care organizations. We'll know a lot more about who within the managed care organizations to go after, what managed care organizations to go after, how to influence the people within the managed care organizations.*

The trend toward increasingly finer segmentation, though, comes with a caveat. Microanalysis could potentially cause companies to lose sight of the big picture if inconsistent drill-down techniques and formats obscure accurate summation of the total market's operation. Decentralized analysis performed without corporate standards and guidelines could lead to a distorted view of the whole or require redundant efforts to restore an overall view.

### Continued Commitment to Customer Satisfaction

Regardless of the degree of a company's original commitment and subsequent adherence to an ongoing process of total quality management, respondents predict that the basic focus on customer needs assessment and satisfaction measurement will persist. As discussed above, pharmaceutical companies must be attentive to understanding and meeting the needs of multiple categories of customers. This is not always easy due to inherently different motivations among these audiences. Perhaps for this reason the patient is often perceived as the ultimate customer to please. When trade-off decisions are necessary, the patient represents a common and "safe" focal point for all of the players involved in health care delivery. The Pharmaceutical Research and Manufacturers Association (PRMA), as well as individual member companies, has increasingly engaged in promotional campaigns to demonstrate how the industry's products have satisfied the specific medical needs of patients.

*Marketing research emphasis in the next five years will be on customers.*

*What we did in the past was marketing research aimed at the customers that we dealt with at that time–physicians–to understand the physicians' needs and the things that they sought from their products and what they needed. Now, we're doing research with all of our customers to find out what their needs are and how we can serve them better.*

The recognized importance of understanding the needs of various categories of external customers is increasing the interactive role that marketing research plays with its internal customer groups. Marketing is not the only internal client interested in customer needs. Business development seeks to clarify specific market demands and to measure current levels of satisfaction as part of the evaluation of new opportunities. Likewise, R&D wants the same information to avoid heavy investment in developing products that will fail to satisfy customer needs or in clinical trials that unknowingly omit measurements or comparisons required to demonstrate a product's ability to satisfy specific needs.

These internal customer needs require the involvement of marketing research earlier and earlier in the process of evaluating new business or clinical opportunities. As a result, the role of marketing research is sometimes enhanced to include a liaison role among the multiple, internal groups who all need valuable customer and market information to reach mutually agreeable decisions.

### Disease Management May Lead to Service Marketing

Disease management is, of course, a comprehensive way of organizing the different components of medical care. Broadly speaking, it unifies traditional medical services (diagnosis, therapy, monitoring, and follow-up), patient support services (counseling, compliance programs, and education), database functions (utilization review), and outcomes measurement. This approach to the delivery of health care is bound to have implications for pharmaceutical sales. For the pharmaceutical industry, disease management has taken on larger significance. These respondents indicate that it has stimulated the broadening of manufacturers' product offerings to include the marketing of services and value-added programs.

Some manufacturers are developing elements of the disease management process and marketing them as revenue-generating services quite apart from the drug products they market. Other manufacturers are developing disease management value-added programs by tying the availability of such services to the sale of their products.

> *Disease management programs are being marketed as disease service programs by pharmaceutical companies now, regardless of whether they involve their products or not. They're getting into whole different types of businesses, and that's because that's where our customers are going.*

At present, primary marketing research is aimed at explaining disease management to upper levels of management. Opinions vary concerning marketing research's future role in disease management. At one extreme, one respondent predicts that there will be no future role for marketing research in disease management after it has been explained to senior management. Most respondents, however, predict an active role for marketing research in guiding the development and marketing of disease management services and measuring their impact just as it has traditionally done for drug products. Still others think marketing research will focus on patient satisfaction.

> *I think we'll be doing less product research and more value-added program type research. I think distinctions in products are going to become less and less important. I think it's "what else can you bring to the party."*

> *So if I can bring a disease management program to you as my customer, that's going to bring you value, and I say, "You know, you have a choice here in these six products. We'd really like you to use [product X] here until someone proves something else is better." Are they going to argue with that? Probably not.*

Another possibility is that the rise of disease management may lead to the use of marketing research as a value-added service or a profit center in its own right. Some manufacturers are offering their own marketing research staffs and resources to conduct studies needed by some of their larger staff model HMO customers. While this use of marketing research can be viewed as value-added service, respondents predict that the sale of marketing research services for profit may not be far behind.

*We'll end up doing more research* [partnering] *which will be between us and managed care organizations. We may well be going out in conjunction with them to research issues that have to do with communication and that kind of thing.*

*I think all the big organizations will be looking to establish partnerships with big managed care customers. What does that partnership look like? I think one of the areas where an organization like this can offer some added value to a managed care organization will be research based. We* [marketing research] *may well, therefore, become part of the added-value program, and it may well be that, "Okay, part of doing this for our product in this formulary position is that we will actually develop the research program which helps you in this way, helps us in this way."*

### Pharmacoeconomics: A New Area for Marketing Research

Pharmacoeconomics, also known as the cost-benefit outcomes analysis of therapeutic interventions, is one of the more visible components of disease management at present. All respondents emphasize its importance and predict that it will continue to be important into the foreseeable future. Determining the market's evaluation and standards for pharmacoeconomic studies is one role marketing research can play. Respondents report that they have qualitatively surveyed managed care organizations to design their pharmacoeconomic studies.

*There is no separate standard in the industry now for doing pharmacoeconomic research. So, in a way, it has to be driven somewhat by the market.*

*I think marketing research can help to identify the type of things that should be looked at in clinical studies. They* [clinical researchers] *move ahead, and they say, "These are the things that we need to show–quality of life and cost and things like that," whereas we can help them up-front identify the things that are important to the decision makers, that they want to see, before they go out and do the studies.*

Respondents predict that, for manufacturers that have not developed distinct pharmacoeconomic units, marketing research departments may be charged with designing and executing pharmacoeconomic studies, or at least managing their design and execution. But even within those companies developing autonomous units, marketing research's involvement with pharmacoeconomic data is inevitable. At the least, a more traditional and familiar role is foreseen for marketing researchers. It will fall upon them to do the research needed to translate pharmacoeconomic data into promotional messages, sales aids, and ad executions and to measure its impact on sales and marketing.

*Some companies may have a designated pharmacoeconomics department, which serves that function. But if they don't, certainly marketing research can do that.*

### Budgets and Head Counts Are Scarce Resources

The 1990s have been marked by the financial pressures placed upon the pharmaceutical industry. Health care reform, political pressure on prices, fewer new product entrants, and other factors have conspired to reduce margins. As a result, the only way to maintain profits has been to control costs. The downsizing experienced by all companies is the most vivid implementation of cost control strategies. Budget reductions closely followed the staff size reductions.

*Competition in the industry is greater. The pressure on individual companies and the external financial pressures on the companies are such that the atmosphere within companies like this is very different now. Issues that have to do with controlling costs, which were not big issues for pharmaceutical industries five to ten years ago, are now such that words like head counts and whatnot are common.*

Furthermore, respondents predict that the head count reductions are not finished. One predicts that R&D will be the next area reduced. He is joined by other respondents in cautioning that marketing research, which has not yet felt the full effect of downsizing, will also be a target for cost containment. The obvious implication of the head count and budget reductions is that marketing research has had and will continue to have fewer resources available to meet management's increasing information needs.

*The first thing that went is corporate staff. The second thing that goes is the sales force. The third thing that's going to go in the next round is going to be R&D. The corporate staff is the easiest. It's the hardest to put a sense on what value they have.*

*Sales is next because they're probably overstaffed because every-body else was. They're going to find that they can't afford to do all of the things that they want to do. So I think R&D is sort of next.*

*Management is going to demand more* [cuts]. *Pharmaceutical companies are shrinking in size. They're reducing their marketing research functions.*

Since the moratorium on health care reform, the budget crunch has eased somewhat. Respondents report that their most recent budgets have grown and that they are doing more projects than ever before. But, even though budgets may have grown, these resources are stretched thin. In the past, marketing research was given budget and personnel resources sufficient to study physician segments. Now, the same efforts must be distributed across multiple segments, including patients, managed care and hospital pharmacists, physicians, nurses, and administrators. The increase in budgets, though, has not been proportional to the increase in segments; thus resources are stretched beyond their limits. This trend, too, is expected to continue into the foreseeable future. As a result, respondents claim that they have to be more fiscally responsible.

*Personally, I know I scrutinize decisions on expenditures more closely than I did three or four or five years ago.*

### Time Is also a Precious Commodity

More than ever before, it seems, there is simply not enough time. This may be because there are fewer hands to do the increasing volume of work demanded of marketing research. Or it may be because the world is simply moving at a faster pace.

*The industry is moving faster, and we need to move faster with things, to provide results faster.*

Whatever the reasons, one of the most visible effects of the time crunch is the need to turn marketing research studies around more quickly than was true in the past. For the most part, this requirement is presently being met by pushing the system to its limits. Studies are simply being done faster by overtaxing existing resources and by reducing the time devoted to data collection by reducing sample sizes, asking respondents for less information, and paying higher honoraria to respondents.

*We have not gotten into too many situations yet where we can't do the research because we can't get it done in time to influence the decision. But what it does do is it puts a big premium on our information technology to be able to manage the data quickly. In other words, from the time that somebody requests a study until we can get it into the field, that time has to shorten. We have to be able to pull our list of physicians almost instantaneously. We have to be able to design our questionnaires very quickly and get them out in the field. It puts a responsibility on our suppliers. We tend to narrow our number of suppliers because we know who can do this quickly and who can do it reliably. So that's where we save our time right now.*

But, in some cases, studies have been foregone because their results could not be obtained in time to have an impact on the decisions to be made. Still, it appears, decision making without the benefit of marketing research is more the exception. Rather than resulting from a conscious decision that marketing research is unneeded, it is often the result of unforeseen events or needs, poor planning, or inattention due to competing demands. Respondents predict that internal clients will wait if they must because the consequences of a wrong decision are simply too severe.

*I think people, if they can, will wait because the downside of getting it wrong is going to be so much bigger than decisions of that type five years ago.*

Another casualty of the time crunch is that there is less time for staff development. As will be discussed, the lack of resources in the face of increased demand requires marketing research personnel to be even more efficient, more productive, and more versatile. This requires ongoing staff development so that personnel can make better use of state-of-the-art tools and methods. Respondents report that the lack of time, more than financing, is an obstacle preventing staff development.

### Geographic Focus Affects Both Structure and Function

The importance of effective and successful market participation at global, national, and regional levels has created basic structural issues for many companies. Essentially, it comes down to a question of centralization versus decentralization of marketing research functions to support marketing efforts for different geographies. Each iteration of restructuring or reengineering is, in part, an attempt to design the ideal organization for implementing the charge "Think globally, act locally."

According to these respondents, regionalization has more tactical than strategic implications. For others, the issue is as simple as waiting to see whether fee-for-service or managed care (and which form of managed care) dominates in one region or another.

*I think regionalization will be much more of a tactical issue.*

*Regionalization is effectively a nice shorthand term for which HMO is going to win in which part of the country to be the dominant market. As a consequence of that, the regionalization will be very much more the tactical issues.*

All indications are that efforts will be increasingly dedicated to understanding smaller and smaller pieces of geography. Marketing research support is and will be required at varying geographic levels, and the marketing research function will continue to experience reorganizations. Coordination and synthesis of secondary data resources, primary research projects, and analytical reports is the key to developing successful marketing plans and, ultimately, to realizing the maximum benefits from the budgetary resources committed. Many companies will be involved in the ongoing pursuit of the structure that best facilitates this coordination and synthesis over the next five years.

*I think we're probably going to look at things on a more regional basis too. Like look at different areas of the country and see if we need to sell our products differently on the West Coast than we do in the South.*

### Marketing Research Must Have a Business Orientation

Just as changes in health care have affected the way pharmaceutical companies sell their products, the orientation of marketing research has to change accordingly. The first change, according to these respondents, is that any proposed marketing research must pass the test that it has the potential to influence decision making. Research to confirm decisions that have already been made and research that cannot be completed in time to influence decisions may not be done at all. Thus, marketing research is required to be action oriented upon initiation.

*I think a lot of times in the past research was done to confirm decisions that were already made rather than used to make decisions. We don't do that anymore. If a decision has already been made, we won't go out and do research to tell them, "Yes, you made the right decision." We won't do any research unless we know what decision rests on the research.*

*If product managers want us to do something, we'll sit down and interview them and find out what the information is that they need and what decisions they are going to make when they have that information and do they really need to do a piece of research to make that decision.*

Respondents also report that marketing research is now required to be less product oriented and more business or issue oriented. Illustrative of this emphasis is a recent organizational name change. The former International Pharmaceutical Marketing Research Group (IPMRG) is now known as the Pharmaceutical Business Intelligence Research Group (PBIRG). Many position titles and department names within companies also reflect this expanded function. The line between primary marketing research and intelligence gathering is not easily drawn any longer. In keeping with this orientation, it is said that traditional research such as that aimed at simply analyzing attributes, tracking product movement, or measuring awareness, for example, can no longer be supported by the limited budgets and manpower available, unless it is related to key marketing issues.

*We do issue-orientated research. We don't just do research to find out what's happening in awareness and usage and those same kind of traditional studies that we did in the past which was sort of research for research's sake. But because of the facts, the constraints on the business, constraints on resources, we must do research that's issue oriented.*

*Issues related to the strategy of the brand or the business are studied. They don't have to be small issues. They could be big issues. But we aren't just going to go out and find out what's the awareness level today, unless it's a problem, unless we have some reason to believe that there's something that needs to be changed about it.*

Pharmaceutical marketing is said to be increasingly involved with business-to-business marketing and selling. As a result, these marketing researchers say more of the requests to which they respond deal with business analysis or studies aimed at resolving specific issues. Examples of the business decisions marketing research is being asked to evaluate include acquisition, licensing, and comarketing opportunities. There is also need for a good understanding of the capabilities and competencies that a company can bring to a potential partnership. It is anticipated that these needs will be even more prevalent through the year 2000.

> *The external change in the market has to do with, as I see it, managed care. We are going to be much more of a business-to-business type of business. Those are more of the relationships that we have.*

In part, the emphasis on having a business outlook is fueled by the fact that more product markets are becoming commodity markets and require a different approach. Dealing with multisource or therapeutically equivalent products has forced companies into more creative business arrangements and contracts. Pharmaceutical manufacturers are looking at unique business opportunities and value-added services rather than tweaking product-oriented strategies. Thus, the information needs of the future will go well beyond the traditional marketed product focus on features and benefits.

> *It depends on the type of products that you're dealing with. If you're dealing with products that are multisource or therapeutic equivalent or whatever, then it's much more of a business-to-business focus and less of a focus on individuals.*

> *Take more of a business outlook on things because a lot of these markets are becoming more commodity markets. That's a different type of business.*

When products are unique, single source, or patent protected, it is predicted that there will be continued demand for many of the traditional kinds of studies. But many of the new products to be launched over the next five years are expected to differ significantly from those of the past. They will originate with genetic engineering and recombinant technology, for example. Or they will penetrate therapeutic areas not previously amenable to pharmacological approaches. For these kinds of products, both traditional product-oriented and business/issue-oriented research will be required.

> *Products that are going to be coming along are going to be unlike many that are out there right now. There's going to be a real premium on the ability to evaluate the business potential of something that our customers have very little experience in dealing with.*

One implication of the need for this sort of information is that marketing research is viewed as a repository of information on a variety of topics and may be considered the expert on specific markets or issues related to brand strategy (e.g., reimbursement obstacles). It is up to marketing research to synthesize the information from all of its activities. It is expected to play an active/proactive role by identifying anything that affects markets and brands. This role requires knowledge and understanding of the company's strategic direction to provide a framework and perspective for meaningful analysis. In general, this expectation cannot be met through traditional marketing research alone but must involve business/competitive intelligence as well. Reviewing the literature, attending industry conferences, attending FDA review sessions, searching on-line databases, working the field with detail reps, meeting with medical consulting/opinion leader boards, and contracting with external intelligence and marketing research consultants are all among the methods employed by marketing researchers as a means for gathering information on competitors and issues.

> *As marketing research people, we are charged with having an understanding of everything in the environment that can affect the success of our business. It's up to us to synthesize everything we get from all of the activities that we do and say these are the impacts on our markets and on our brands.*

> *The marketing research person is looked upon as a source of information on any number or variety of topics. You have to be sort of a depository of that information. You become more of an active/proactive participant that is sort of the expert on the market and the environment.*

In support of this role, marketing researchers commonly are active participants on multidisciplinary teams. Respondents claim that the impetus for this involvement is tied to changes in the marketplace, which increase the risk of business failure. Simply launching a new product is not enough. The information marketing research can provide reduces the risk of failure when introduced early into the process of drug development and clinical testing.

> *A lot of our effort has been directed toward working with clinical trials people and incorporating different types of measures into those clinical trials, whether they be economic measures or measures of different outcomes or endpoints that are needed. We no longer can afford to have a drug come to Phase III or be launched and then realize that we didn't do a trial with endpoints that the market needs to see. We can't afford that anymore.*

*I think the whole role of marketing research in relation to clinical R&D has certainly changed. I think it really all comes back to changes in the marketplace and the changes and the pressures on pharmaceutical companies. All of the changes in the marketplace have put additional pressures on R&D to develop either products that have significant advantages or something that can be marketable. Now they need our input to tell them what the best candidates are or how to manage the development process in order to enhance the marketability of the product.*

Adding a business/issue-orientation to marketing research's responsibilities and knowing when also to rely on traditional studies poses a significant challenge. Respondents acknowledge the increase in technical sophistication needed. Some companies have responded by changing the criteria used to select marketing research personnel, placing a premium on business education and acumen. They hire M.B.A.s from top schools and give them on-the-job training in marketing research and the pharmaceutical industry. What hasn't changed is the "pass-through" phenomenon. Marketing research is still considered a stepping stone to positions in product management or other line functions to which many staffers aspire. Their tenure in marketing research is unlikely to be more than two to three years.

One of the benefits to marketing research of being a pass-through function is that as corporate climbers who have served time in marketing research early in their careers move to the top corporate echelons, they will, theoretically, have more appreciation for the capabilities and value of marketing research. They will understand the contributions that can be made at both tactical and strategic levels. Consequently, marketing research should be more respected, involved, and relied on by these managers.

Unfortunately, when pass through is pervasive, marketing research suffers from a lack of experienced researchers. This is all the more telling as the technical demands on marketing research increase. Additionally, marketing research is continually robbed of its best talent. A few companies have enjoyed stability at the director and manager levels, while others have experienced nearly constant turnover. These respondents claim that the best structure is a mix of permanent and pass-through staffing. The permanent staffers acquire valuable experience and expertise, while the pass throughs introduce fresh blood and fresh perspectives.

### Process Research Is More Prevalent

Historically, most pharmaceutical marketing research has been of an applied nature, meaning that it applies well-known methods to tactical or strategic product marketing issues. This can be contrasted with basic research, which seeks to understand the processes underlying the functioning of some system or to develop the technology needed to study or influence the behavior of such systems. The pervasive changes in the delivery of health care have caused pharmaceutical marketing research to depart from its traditional emphasis on applied research. Some respondents predict that less effort will be devoted to the tactical research more common to this industry.

> *Maybe three or four years ago, things may have been approached a little bit more in a piecemeal fashion. We have a journal ad and you need to go measure the effectiveness of the journal ad. We have a competitive product coming out and you need to go through a competitive analysis. Whatever. But I think those days are gone, of people doing structured marketing plans, and a lot of data that used to be collected all the time, the thick reports, and the standard journal ad tests and all that stuff, the companies that are focusing there primarily with their marketing research department are being eliminated or reduced.*

Other respondents revise this prediction to state that such traditional research will always be needed but added the research of a more basic nature will be done to understand the processes currently operating in pharmaceutical markets. If this latter group is correct in predicting that the accommodation of basic or process-oriented research will expand rather than replace current activities, there will be even more pressure on the finite resources devoted to marketing research. In any event, it is clear that there will be more emphasis on basic marketing research than in the past.

> *I believe we're confronted with this big black box called managed care right now, which none of us really feel confident that we understand. We have to understand those processes before we can turn back and do the more kinds of traditional things that marketing research has done.*

> *At the end of the day, the process for getting our product goal was fairly simple. We went and talked to a doctor, the doctor said, "Oh, that's interesting," and if he or she could remember it two days later when the patient came in, you sold the product, period. But the actual customer base now is employing more processes to make these decisions competently. The trend to understand what those processes are, I think, is evident.*

*You're really trying to monitor and stay on top of how health care is being delivered and what's happening in the market in terms of the decision makers. Not so much tactical or applied research on how we're going to price our product or position our product, but just trying to let the people in upper management know and in our sales organization know what in the world is going on out there with companies buying other companies and why they're doing that and who our new customers are.*

The need for this process research is not tied just to the changes in health care delivery. It is also blamed on the failure of secondary data to keep pace with the information needs of pharmaceutical marketing researchers. The audits remain almost solely product movement and physician oriented. But, as respondents have made clear, current information needs are oriented to other business issues and other segments of the health care industry. There is a paucity of audit data tracking drugs by formulary approval, product movement through managed care organization (MCO) physicians or pharmacy benefit managers (PBMs), and patients' influence on product movement, for example.

*While we have more data than we could ever possibly use on doctors' prescribing and dispensing pharmaceuticals, we don't have enough data on formulary structure and how many prescriptions are dispensed under a controlled formulary versus a noncontrolled formulary or one where there's preferred status or not. We have some basic data about the plans and how much business goes through the plans, but those sources are not yet nearly as well developed as the sources we have had in the past for physicians.*

*We have to understand what the hospital needs. We have to understand what the managed care plan needs. We have to understand what the payer needs. What the PBM needs. And how we can then use that information about their needs and their goals to work out some kind of way to develop a marketing or selling plan that fits those needs so that we can get our business moved forward by servicing our customers' needs.*

Finally, as in other developments, there is an increased need for marketing research to be flexible and ever adaptable. The processes that are the focus of the basic research under investigation are still evolving and are expected to evolve for some time. After having done a few studies, it may be tempting to think that we have figured out the system, but this is a dangerous posture. The system is likely to continue changing while the data collected by these studies is being analyzed. Thus, marketing researchers must continue gathering data and questioning their assumptions until a return to equilibrium has been documented by the lack of further change.

*Things are changing so fast that a year from now, where are things going to be? They're not going to be the way they are now based on what the people that we spoke to are saying.*

*I think it's constantly changing. I'm not sure we now understand at this point what the process is, but I think the process is changing.*

## CONCLUSIONS

It is obvious that sorting out the full implications of the factors affecting marketing research through the year 2000 is not an easy process. As is true in any system, these factors are inexorably linked. When they point to the same needs resulting in common implications, the task of predicting the future is easier. But often their implications are at odds with one another, and it may be too soon to predict which factors will dominate the future.

Furthermore, marketing research services the needs of managers of all levels and in all functional units. As such, it is logical that it will lag behind management in responding to the changes in the marketplace. As management adapts to the new environment, its information needs will become apparent and will be articulated to marketing research. At present, primary marketing researchers are just beginning to field the requests that result from environmental changes. It must be noted, however, that this view is at odds with the contention that marketing research should be proactive in leading the way. It is also at odds with the fact that so-called marketing research departments are doing much more than strict marketing research.

Adding to the prediction problem is the fact that the health care and pharmaceutical industries are in the midst of change. Predictions made at this time suffer in that they may be based on unstable data. The concrete trends and tendencies pointing the direction back to equilibrium may not be evident or may not yet have emerged. Still, in response to this observation, these respondents claim that some of the implications of these factors have become concrete and that reliable predictions can be made.

### Samples Will Be More Diverse and Smaller

The need for more diverse samples derives from the need to match the changes in marketing's audiences. The prediction that samples will be smaller is a function of many factors, including the declining resources and the fact that the universe of respondents in some of the segments targeted by marketing is small. Because some of the universes are small, there will be an urgent need to develop strategies for sample access. As small segments are increasingly studied, they burn out on doing research and access diminishes.

> *I think that there's going to be less of these people from a sampling point of view. Getting to them will be more difficult. I think they will likely become more skeptical about market research.*

> *There's got to be an increasing challenge to reach people in primary research. Everybody is going to be doing more and more of it, and the targets are going to become fewer and fewer. You're going to be challenged to get to those people.*

In turn, the recognition that, in the future, samples will be smaller leads to a call for the use and development of methods suited to small-sample research. Complicating the problem is the fact that marketing research is still going to need information on decision makers' motivations, product and service needs and evaluation, evaluation of promotional materials, promotion response, awareness levels, etc.

> *I think the other thing is while the concept of the research remains the same, we must learn to develop new methodologies, new ways of getting to the customers because our concept is, "Yes, we're still the same. We have to understand our customers' needs and figure out how to meet them." But the fact that we have a whole new set of customers that we have to address brings up issues of how to get to them and how best to ask them questions and whatnot.*

> *You couldn't get the numbers if you wanted to because trying to interview these people is very difficult.*

### Databases Make Primary Research Easier

As has been discussed, the increasing availability of databases has contributed to the pharmaceutical industry's information overload. To an extent, some of the primary research done to describe the market has been and will continue to be obviated by the analysis of database information. Even some of the primary research aimed at explaining and predicting market behavior will be supplanted by database manipulations, although this is less common. But the availability and analysis of database information is expected to increase–rather than reduce–the demand for primary research. As marketing researchers gain more insight into market operations, they expect new questions to emerge. It is further expected that answering these questions will require primary research.

> *Having data available allows us to go the next step and say, "Now that we know this, let's examine it, let's evaluate it, and it may raise questions that we can now spin-off new research projects from." Now we have an insight that we didn't have before, and it either raises a question or helps us answer something that we need to go further on.*

Databases will also refocus the type of primary research that can be done. In many ways, the database information has made primary research easier. Sampling is probably the first way in which databases have an affect on primary research. As they are used for target marketing, the databases provide lists from which to sample respondents. More importantly, the incidence of qualified respondents increases when the databases are composed of targeted customers. In the past, all physicians in their respective populations were listed, resulting in a great deal of wasted effort.

> *I think the availability of databases has also made the kind of research we do more productive because we can very easily recruit and target, for research, specific subsets of physicians or specific customers who we want answers from.*

> *It certainly takes a lot more time to do it* [sample] *by screening, and more money. The accuracy of your screening is improved by having, for example, a pharmacy records database. You know exactly how many prescriptions were dispensed by that physician for a certain brand or category. If you have to screen to get physicians, you get a perception of prescribing.*

> *Before you might not even have been able to do some analyses because you could never screen physicians accurately enough to know which ones were affiliated with which health care plans, etc.*

Primary research can also be done more easily because interview time can be reduced now that some questions which are traditionally asked can be obtained from databases. This could reduce the time and expense of conducting primary research. More often than not, however, it simply frees marketing researchers to use the survey time for other purposes. Thus, in the future, primary research studies will either be shorter or more complex and creative. The former has budgetary implications, while the latter has implications for marketing research personnel.

> *If you're able through a database, ScripTrac Plus or whatever, to identify what your target audience is, and you know what questions you want to ask that target audience, then you've got everything. You've got your audience, and you've got your questions, versus before you needed to identify who they were, and then you had to identify what was driving them, and then you needed to ask them questions and direct your strategy. So in that way, it's become easier.*

> *I think you can do more things if you're creative. There are people who are into the psychometric segmentation now using a lot of these physician-level databases. So you can either buy into that or not buy into that, but I think with the existence of these databases, it creates the possibility to spend your time doing a lot more creative things, doing a lot more potentially value-added things.*

Another way in which primary research has been made easier is by merging database information with survey research information. This has the potential to increase the quality of primary research in two ways. First, audit quality data can be substituted for perceptual data. This is especially valuable when actual behavior can be substituted for measures of perceived behavior. Second, as addressed above, information merged from a database will obviate the need to pose some questions. The interview time thus saved can be used to gather added information, enabling the research to achieve more depth, breadth, or enhanced model building.

> *You can merge database information with your survey research information to replace information gathered in the survey, reducing the time you ask those kinds of questions, and ask different questions.*

### Need to Assess Quality of Databases

One of the more subtle implications of database proliferation is the need to verify the validity of the information. There is a tendency to accept the information in databases as hard fact. Often it deserves this status. But there are times when it does not. Some databases are merely a compilation of perceptual data and, therefore, are not factual at all.

*At present, a lot of the data can't be confirmed, and sources are questionable. Someone is going to have to get a handle on this first.*

More commonly, databases present factual snapshots of the market at one point in time. And like old photographs, they become old and out-dated. The individuals on whom data has been archived drop out of prac-tice, change organizations, or change positions within organizations. They change specialties or move to other areas of the country. Their behaviors change. They stop prescribing the products they used when the database information was gathered and switch to other products. Each of these phenomena increases the amount of error in a database. While any one of these sources may introduce only a small amount of error, together they combine for a significant amount of total error. And this cannot be consid-ered a comprehensive list of error types. Yet decisions, both marketing and marketing research, are being made based on the information in these databases without any attempt to judge the validity of that information.

Developing protocols for updating or refreshing the databases is necessary but not sufficient. Given the insidious nature of the error in databases, meth-ods and expertise must be developed for assessing the validity of, identifying the inaccuracies in, and correcting errors in database information.

### Qualitative Research Will Increase in Importance

According to these respondents, the volume of group depth interviews (GDIs) and individual depth interviews (IDIs) has increased and will continue to increase. Some report that their reliance on qualitative research has increased at the expense of quantitative studies. Others claim that while they are doing more qualitative research, they are also doing more quantitative research. They maintain that volume of research overall has increased and that the mix of qualitative and quantitative is the same.

*I don't know that it's shifted in one direction or another, but we're doing a lot more than we ever used to do. I think we're relying more and more on primary research than we did in the past. I've been in the department for eight years, and we do a tremendous amount more on both the qualitative and quantitative sides than we ever did before.*

Whether the proportion of qualitative studies has risen or not, all respondents agree that its volume will continue to rise. This rise responds to the need to use smaller samples, less time, smaller budgets, and a focus on process research. It also responds to the fact that pharmaceutical marketing's new audiences often come from very small populations. Short of doing a census, there simply is no opportunity to compile large samples. This problem is compounded when there is a desire to segment these audiences into more precise targets. Nowhere is this more true than with PBMs and within the managed care market. The number of MCOs is small in total. But when it is to be segmented into staff-model HMOs, IPAs, and PPOs, the population is stretched thin. It is stretched more thinly still if these segments are to be further subsegmented, for example into those with closed or open formularies. Even when quantitative measures are sought within such small samples, the data must be viewed as yielding qualitative-level information.

*Right now, we're stuck almost entirely with qualitative research because there just aren't enough managed care respondents, and their decision making is very concentrated.*

Time, as has been noted, is scarce. Management's need for marketing research information is totally contingent on when that information is received. The best information is worthless when received too late (or, for that matter, too early). Time pressures influence the volume of qualitative research in yet another way. The pace of change in the marketplace must be matched with the pace at which research can be conducted. The fact that the pharmaceutical marketplace is changing from moment to moment demands the short time frames possible with qualitative research. The possibility that market processes will change between the time data is collected and results are reported is a very real source of error. And the probability of error increases as the duration of a research project increases. Qualitative research can provide insights, if not final reports, more quickly. Strategy often begins to evolve "behind the glass."

*I think that the speed at which the market has changed over the last couple of years also favors qualitative.*

The need to understand the processes in the marketplace also enhances the need for qualitative research. It has long been known that qualitative research is capable of discovering and explaining market behavior. It is, in a sense, descriptive by nature. By contrast, quantitative methods obtain precise measurements to be used for prediction and/or hypothesis testing.

The less one knows about any particular phenomenon of interest, the higher the need for qualitative research and the less able one is to design quantitative studies. Given the new processes emerging in the health care market, the questions pharmaceutical marketers need to have answered are qualitative in nature. Only when these processes reach equilibrium and are well known will quantitative research become more feasible.

> *You really have to question, "Do I really know what's going on?" And it forces you to learn more and more about the whole environment that things are happening in. I think this favors qualitative research in part because it helps to give you the sense of where things are.*

> *You're sort of taking people through, "How is it that you do business now? What are the things that you're deciding on? How would this impact on your business?" It's very qualitative. So the type of business that we're doing also tends to lend itself more toward qualitative.*

Even though GDIs and IDIs are well suited to the current environment, these respondents clearly indicate that the status quo is unacceptable. They question the small, nonrandom sampling methods and exhibit all too common traditional lack of faith in the direct questions posed in qualitative settings. Whether unfounded or not, some respondents call for the development of new and improved qualitative methods.

> *Qualitative has its own problems. It's sort of the level of meaning that you're dealing with. Is it top of mind because it sounds good at the time and that's what your respondents are telling you, or is it true? How do you get them down to the level of, "Well, this is actually the stuff that I make my decisions based on."*

> *You start off with paying these people. What is normal human nature? Normal human nature is "I'll tell you what it is I think you want to hear." It's normal psychology.*

More important, perhaps, is the finding that the growth in qualitative research is, in part, due to the development and use of new and different qualitative methods. Qualitative "crafting" of positions and messages is the new buzzword. Additionally, these respondents report the use of new psychological techniques and the mixing of qualitative and quantitative methods. It is clear that qualitative research is becoming more innovative, is becoming more creative, and is evolving through the use of new methods. As a result, it has been hypothesized that it is getting more marketing research attention, which makes it seem as if more is being done.

> *The trend is more and more toward doing more than just testing sales aids. We're spending a lot more time with new techniques in crafting the positioning and crafting the message behind the products using some new techniques. More reliance on linguistic research, more reliance on image research, things that can get you more into brand character and brand personality than ever before. We're also doing brand personality work a lot as part of the initial positioning and message development work.*

> *You make the task you want him to do so difficult that he can't figure out how to put the spin on it that he thinks you'd like. So you get him to do things. Get him to play with cards. Things like conjoint; it's sort of the same basis. You get him to do something that gets to a level of where he has to resort to his own basic intuition because it's just too hard to play games anymore. Even in qualitative research where you don't actually want to go for that level of quantification you can do the same type of thing. You give him a task that is, in essence, so difficult for him to do that he can't just tell you what it is you want to hear.*

### Quantitative Methods Must Adapt

The need for primary quantitative research will remain as strong in the future as it has been in the past, but the methods used and the deliverables must change to meet the needs of the changing marketplace. Virtually all of the factors identified as influencing marketing research have implications for quantitative methods. In the future, primary quantitative research methods will need to:

- Rely on new data collection tools which enable respondents to provide the data required to take advantage of new statistical technology
- Integrate smoothly with information obtained from secondary sources, i.e., databases
- Model decision making based on the changing health care delivery processes (e.g., disease management and pharmacoeconomics) in the marketplace
- Integrate the unique objective functions and the decision processes of each target segment into a single decision or prediction of behavior while retaining segment differences in support of target marketing

- Be more efficient, providing results more quickly based on smaller samples
- Provide business-oriented information rather than data.

## Quantitative Research Takes Too Long

Reducing the time required is one of the first adaptations that quantitative methods must make. It has already been emphasized that qualitative methods benefit from the fact that their time requirements are more consistent with changing market dynamics and management's demands. There is no question, based on these interviews, that the unique assets of quantitative research are still valued, but only if they are realized in time to improve the quality of decision making.

> *Things are changing very quickly. To take a snapshot in time with a big quantitative study takes six months to do it. Then in that six more months, things have changed so much that you might not feel you want to go back and use that as your stake in the ground.*

> *One of the problems, however, [with quantitative] is you don't have time to put out a 300 physician survey and wait for all of the things to get back because the questions that you're asking when you design a survey in November and when you finally get the stuff back in April, it isn't relevant anymore. So how do you deal with that? So you go to qualitative.*

Increasingly, these respondents say that they are turning to research consultants who can compress the amount of time devoted to all stages of quantitative studies.[2] To deliver on these demands, primary quantitative researchers will have to define their clients' needs and wants accurately and then develop the means to deliver what is needed and wanted more quickly.

## Pricing Research Must Avert Costly Mistakes

Pricing research has taken on added importance, largely because of the political climate. Throughout most of the 1980s, price increases were used as the fastest and easiest tools to increase profits. In the early 1990s, it became apparent that health care reform was going to control this tool unless the industry found the means to control itself. Thus, determining the prices at which new products are introduced takes on added importance.

There will not be opportunities to raise the prices of new products introduced at prices less than the market will bear. On the other hand, public outrage at products introduced at prices perceived as extremely high invites government intervention.

> *How you're pricing your product and how somebody else is pricing it. That sort of price warfare that goes on, which in this industry, five years ago, nobody talked about. If they did, it was sort of in a general sense. If you studied product attributes and you said, "Well, efficacy is important and safety is important, side effects are important, convenience is now less important, and down below everything else is price." Because nobody knew what price was. The guy who was paying for it had no control over it. The guy who was ordering it didn't know what the price was, and the guy who was paying for it at the end had no control over any of that. It was sort of a wonderful, nice system.*

The market forces outlined above have placed more pressure on pricing research, and that pressure has revealed an undercurrent of dissatisfaction with the methods employed and the results delivered by pricing studies. One reason why pricing research has been historically unsatisfying is because it needed to focus on physicians who neither knew nor cared about the prices of the products they prescribed. Yet they controlled the demand for these products. In more recent years, pricing research has also failed to focus on the emergent segments controlling demand, i.e., hospital pharmacists and managed care decision makers. These emergent segments will continue to be important in the next five years and beyond. But within this period, patients themselves will emerge as the next segment to control demand. Thus, primary research must continually adapt to obtain pricing information from a variety of decision-making segments.

> *When you set a price, there are more people that you have to talk to than the physician. My feeling is that pricing was always very difficult because the physicians didn't know the price. It's becoming easier now because physicians are becoming more aware of the pricing of drugs. But it's more difficult because of the other people.*

A second potential source of dissatisfaction with pricing research seems to center on the methods themselves. These interviews reveal that internal clients are skeptical about the validity of pricing study results. They have concerns about the way in which pricing questions are asked, the samples surveyed, and those needing to be surveyed. As a result, these internal clients, apparently, are led to establish prices based more on management judgment than on hard data.

> *The question that our product managers are starting to ask now is, "If you go into a managed care decision maker and present him or her with a set of prices for this product, don't you expect that they're going to pick the lowest price because they want you to come back with that contracting strategy?" I think there's a great deal of skepticism that we can get true answers without really realizing that we're influencing the decision by asking the questions.*

> *I think we haven't really made a big contribution in the area of pricing. Part of it is that upper management doesn't really believe in pricing studies. They make pricing decisions based on sort of a gut feel. But I think the other issue is again the market is not as homogenous as it used to be, so it's difficult to do traditional conjoint-type pricing studies. I'm not sure that we've figured out really how to do good pricing studies in marketing research.*

A third potential source of dissatisfaction may be that, at present, state-of-the-art pricing studies fail to recommend a specific price. However, the users of pricing research must accept some of the responsibility for this failing. Without added information, pricing studies, by definition, will be unable to recommend specific price points.

According to economic theory, prices should be set relative to corporate objectives. The information to be gathered in pricing studies depends on those objectives. Little information is needed to price so as to maximize share, as the lowest feasible price will accomplish this goal. Revenue maximization requires an estimate of demand elasticity, for which pricing research is needed. But, elasticity in itself will only point in the direction of a high or low price. It only makes a specific price point recommendation when the feasible price range has firm upper and lower bounds. Then, however, either the highest or the lowest price will be recommended when elasticity information is taken by itself. The lack of a precise price recommendation has often been unsatisfying and has fueled skepticism about the worth of pricing studies.

The recommendation of one specific optimal price requires internal and competitive information that is not readily accessible. The ability to recommend a specific price from within a feasible range is consistent with the goal of profit maximization. Economic theory states that the profit maximizing price occurs where marginal revenue equals marginal cost. Present studies, by documenting the demand curve (from which price elasticity is obtained), provide the means to obtain marginal revenue. But it is only possible to obtain marginal cost from a curve relating total cost to various levels of production, i.e., the total cost curve. This internal information is usually unknown to the users of pricing studies and may only be obtainable with considerable effort. To make matters worse, pricing studies should be done in competitively simulated markets, and this requires total cost curves for competitive products, too.

In the future, a better partnership is indicated between those charged with doing pricing studies and those wanting to use the results. The users of pricing studies must provide more internal information. Those conducting pricing studies need to take responsibility for three elements in these dynamics. First, they need to understand the economics of pricing. Second, they need to educate users about the internal information the research requires and the deliverables they should expect, given the information that can be provided. Third, they need to develop and employ methods that ask the right questions of the right respondents and are capable of processing both survey and internal information.

### Primary Research Must Better Predict the Future

Just as pricing research has become more important as a result of external forces, the increasing uncertainty surrounding the future configuration of the health care system has increased respondents' focus on primary research's predictive failings. A traditional caveat of any predictive research, whether primary or secondary, is that it may fail to make accurate predictions at the turning points in trends. The present marketplace is all turning points. In spite of all of the technological and database advancements, the pharmaceutical industry is still making predictions in traditional ways. The failure of these methods has become more obvious.

> *I don't want to be able to just say to the marketers, "Here are the segments. This is the way they fall out on the basis of past behavior." What I want to be able to say is, "Here are the segments, and if you say this to them, this is how they'll react." We don't do that terribly well. That's what we should be aiming to do.*

For primary research, another crucial challenge is to improve predictive ability. The quest to link attitudes and past behavior to future behavior has never been satisfied. Micromarketing databases have added to the frustration. Their data, which reports in great detail how individual physicians have been prescribing, seems at odds with what physicians believe they have been doing. It is not clear which is the best marketing target, actual or perceived behavior.

> *I think we haven't been successful in being able to link behavior more closely to attitudes via micromarketing, via the availability of individual prescriber level data. We're able to tell what doctors are doing, but yet when you go and ask them what they're doing, that still isn't the same.*

> *We can say that we know what physicians are doing and here is what they believe about products. It's not making the link between what we know they're doing and what they believe they're doing. That's where we have a disconnect. We don't know why that is.*

Some implications of this dilemma are evident. First, resources must be devoted to the development of new methods capable of predicting behavior from attitudinal and/or perceptual data. Second, marketing researchers and upper management should probably realize that their frustration with predictive methods is probably misplaced. In reality, their frustration probably stems from the inaccuracy of predictions made during periods of disequilibrium. Nevertheless, a third implication for marketing research is the need to develop better predictive methods and procedures for using them during periods of high uncertainty.

Traditionally, these procedures call for identifying the key assumptions underlying predictions and/or the assumptions most subject to uncertainty. Then, marketing research should perform simulations and sensitivity analyses to document the effects of alternative assumptions on the forecasts. When armed with each scenario's likelihood of occurrence as a result of these different assumptions, marketing management can be prepared with a contingency plan for each scenario. Then, as reality begins to unfold, management must have the ability and flexibility to change and adapt quickly by implementing the proper contingency plan.

### Traditional Quantitative Methods Will Still Be Needed

Despite the emphasis placed on the need for adaptation and development of new quantitative methods, it is predicted that there will always be some demand for the approaches employed throughout the last decade. Respondents claim that a portion of the marketing research they do continues in this tradition.

> *We're still doing what we did before in terms of sales aid testing, but it's also looking earlier on.*

First, they explain, they have no complaint with many of these traditional methods and simply need to apply them to new market segments or new issues. Second, for new products, especially those that are unique in some way, respondents still see physicians as the primary decision makers. For these products, physicians rather than PBMs, MCOs, or formularies will direct demand. Because this is traditionally how the market operated, the reasoning goes, it can be studied in traditional ways.

> *If it's unique or first on the market in a new category, then I think you're back to basics and the traditional type of marketing research. The decision maker is still the doctor. Your main focus is the P&T committee, and the key decision maker for use is the physician.*

Third, the view that there will always be a decision-making role for physicians no matter what the class of agents or control from third parties– is also prevalent. In part, this view emanates from the recognition of physicians' important roles in delivering health care services. But this view may also anticipate the ultimate influence that physician organizations will have on the evolution of the health care delivery system.

> *I could never see formularies and treatment protocols getting to the point with the majority of customers where there will never, ever, be a decision for the physician to make on the choice of product. There will always be that decision at the end of the line. Maybe a much more restricted one than there was five years ago, so I don't think traditional [research] will ever go away.*

### Marketing Research Personnel Qualifications Will Change

The increasing demands for different, more complex, and more timely information, coupled with shrinking resources to acquire, analyze, interpret, and apply data, will, according to these respondents, profoundly affect the qualifications of the people who perform marketing research functions. Marketing researchers are being asked to do more, in terms of both volume and expanded involvement in new areas, with fewer people and strained budgets in shorter time frames. And they are being asked to do it better. Clearly, different types of people are going to be required to meet pharmaceutical company needs.

> *I think the role that we're undertaking is becoming too important and too complex to rely on the old "Let's take the sales rep who we think has a little potential, give him a little rotation through marketing research to learn what marketing is all about."*

The traditional use of marketing research as a stepping stone to develop sales people who aspire to product management will no longer be as viable a means for staffing marketing research departments–at least not to the extent that it has been used in the past. The demands being placed on marketing research call for the expertise of more seasoned marketing researchers with longer tenures. Respondents claim that these demands simply cannot be met with former sales reps who begin their marketing research rotations without any marketing research experience or training. Furthermore, the demands on experienced personnel prevent them from training new personnel as much as was the case in the past. Departments may never be 100% staffed with career researchers, but at least a better balance with passthroughs is called for, and the length of time the pass throughs spend in the department must be extended.

> *You can't afford in a time of shrinking resources, human and otherwise, to spend your time constantly training and retraining and retraining and retraining.*

> *Everybody is so caught up in getting their work done and the backlog of work that there's very little time for training and development, particularly the quantitative side.*

> *I don't think it will ever be 100% marketing researchers. I'm not sure I would want it to be 100% career marketing researchers. At some point, you're going to have people developing through to other functions, but it has to be slower than in the past, and the percentage of people moving has to be lower than in the past.*

On-the-job training of marketing research is still seen as the easy part of bringing a new analyst up to speed, especially on the qualitative side. However, according to these respondents, the new job requirements include knowledge and skills that are not easy to teach or learn on the job. The fact that these skills may not currently reside in marketing research departments due to downsizing and turnover means that the ability to provide marketing research, much less train new analysts, is compromised. Thus, ideally, these skills should be in place upon presentation for the job interview.

> *The person that I'm hiring to fill a position is a pharmacist with a Ph.D. in statistics and an advanced degree in marketing research. So there is sort of a whole conglomerate of business and technical skills. The core set of skills that you need to search for to do the type*

*of work that we're talking about is different than it would have been five years ago when all you needed was somebody who sort of understood how physicians reacted to sales aids.*

In the new people they hire, respondents emphasize the need for technical education and training in forecasting methods, statistics, consumer research methods and resources, and competitor/business intelligence methods. In addition, as listed by these respondents, the qualifications and competencies new marketing researchers should have cover a wide variety of areas, including:

- A working knowledge of the health care system *"to understand the context that things are happening in for your product"*
- Analytical skills, defined as the ability to *"see the relationships between things"*
- Verbal and written communications skills because *"as the issues become more complex, communication around those issues becomes more complex"*
- Interpersonal skills sufficient to *"interact with a lot of different levels of people within a lot of different functions within the organization"*
- Computer skills *"because the era of saying, 'Gentlemen, don't use computers' is over. Unless you're in senior management and above, you're not going to get away with that anymore."*

But, the technical competencies of internal marketing research personnel also need to be put into context. Respondents explain that knowing the options in terms of what different techniques can provide, who the experts are who can provide reliable answers, and the limitations of the techniques is more important than being able to execute projects internally. Thus, another required internal skill set deals with the ability to interact with consultants. This set includes interpersonal skills to function in a liaison role between internal clients and outside consultants; communication skills to articulate clearly management's problems/questions/issues and disseminate requests for proposals; business skills to select a proposal based on objective, identified criteria and to negotiate contracts with outside consultants; project (i.e., consultant) management skills; and technical skills to evaluate the quality of the completed project and service. In addition, most internal presentation and use of any research will fall to marketing research analysts and managers. They must be technically competent enough to understand and present an outside consultant's work.

> *It's not so much I can sit down and write a questionnaire as a marketing research analyst or I can design a conjoint study, but it's knowing when I should use it, what I can expect out of it, and who can do it for me. So, if you're talking about what technical skills do we need, I think it's more understanding rather than being able to go out and do it yourself.*

Finally, the marketing researchers of the 21st century need the ability to place all the data and information they are integrating into a business context. Most companies now recognize the need for people who can see the big picture and have the ability to integrate and organize pieces of information to see the relationships among them and their implications for the business of developing and marketing pharmaceutical care. This typically translates to business knowledge in the form of an M.B.A. and/or relevant business experience. The overwhelming need is for people who understand the dynamics of the marketplace and the forces that are interacting to reshape the health care context. A clear understanding of the company's strategic direction and the ability to apply strategic thinking to decision making is also critical.

> *It goes beyond just taking a set of data and reporting the results of a study. It's integrating the results of that study into everything that you know about this marketplace and either your product or your company that's into it. That is more and more what is being demanded of us. We can't just take a set of data tables and say, "Here's what physicians think." It has to be what does that mean in terms of the business decisions that have to be made around this product.*

Pharmaceutical companies with marketing research departments that fail to meet these new knowledge and skill requirements and fail to become integrated team players will be at the mercy of those that can and do.

## Outsourcing Will Increase

The outsourcing of marketing research to consultants has always been the case. Data collection and tabulation have always been outsourced to "field-and-tab" and "watts" houses. For a more complicated or important class of research, study design, analysis, and reporting, as well as data collection and tabulation, have also been outsourced to full-service marketing researchers. For the most complicated, most important, and most visible research projects, study design and execution, as well as consulting with upper management on the study's strategic implications, have been outsourced.

Just as the requirements for internal marketing research personnel have been restated, the future will not mean business as usual for outside consultants either. Respondents predict that the form of outsourcing described above will increase, becoming even more pervasive due to fewer in-house personnel and more demands on their time. It may well be that almost no studies will be designed and analyzed internally. If so, there will be a greater need for full-service marketing research consultants and less need for field-and-tab houses. Marketing research consultants will be asked to provide more full-service support to their clients, support that goes well beyond just data collection and cross tabulation. On the front end, consultants will be responsible for selection of study methodology and study design. Once the data is in hand, consultants will analyze it, report it, interpret it, present it, and recommend actions. The education and training on how to use data is a void that consultants will be asked to fill.

Furthermore, clients are looking for people who can provide these services with little or no direction. This represents a whole new level of expertise, requiring improved knowledge and skills exceeding those available internally. The emphasis on information rather than data and on having a business focus will lead to increased reliance on marketing researchers who already function as consultants or can quickly, easily, and successfully make the transition from marketing research "supplier" to marketing research "consultant."

> *What you're looking for again, is people who you can farm out some of that information to so the person who's doing the interviewing also brings some expertise and some knowledge and some insights to help you sort of process through it, too.*

To provide these new levels of service effectively, the client/supplier relationship will have to become more intimate than ever before. The present system of outsourcing, involving a variety of client-consultant relationships, has served the industry well and can continue to do so. But new forms of contractual relationships can also be explored. Short-term, project-oriented agreements that place individual consultants on-site have been commonplace in many companies and will probably continue. One new model might be to enter into long-term exclusive contracts with consultant firms to provide primary marketing research services on a therapeutic-area-by-therapeutic-area basis. This is analogous to the normal *modus operandi* for advertising agencies. The present supply of required expertise on the consultant side available to meet the potential demand for such arrangements is limited. Thus, pharmaceutical companies might gain a competitive edge through such exclusive arrangements.

A second possible model is the outsourcing of total marketing research departments to independent firms placing their consultants on-site full-time in their clients' facilities. To be successful in this capacity, though, consultant firms must be more than the full-service primary marketing research firms they are at present. They must be equipped to meet all the demands for both primary and secondary research, and they must come with pharmaceutical business knowledge and internal corporate operations experience equivalent to that presently demanded of internal marketing research personnel. These comprehensive qualifications are rare, if they exist at all. To date, there have only been two or three experiments with this model. These experiments have not yet been evaluated, so there are no predictions that they will become more widespread in the future.

### Marketing Research Must Take Responsibility for Its Own Future

Given the conclusions offered about primary research's ability to make predictions under uncertain conditions, there is a certain irony to the challenge of this project's undertaking, i.e., to predict the future of primary marketing research. While it is known that the factors identified will definitely affect primary marketing research in the logical ways predicted by this panel of experienced players and observers, the ultimate outcomes are not always clear. Even these respondents say they do not know when equilibrium will be restored or what the picture of primary marketing research will be at that point.

> *I think the general points that have been made with regard to different customer types, issues to do with managed care and all those sorts of issues. Those general directions, I think, are pretty soundly based. I think the implications for market research and all of those implication-type issues that we've discussed, I think it's fair to say we don't know exactly what those implications are.*

Ultimately, respondents agree that primary marketing research should take command of its own future. Other writers on this topic have called for paradigm shifts and quality producing research rather than quality control research. The findings reported here support their conclusions. Their efforts as well as this one sound the warnings being issued by internal clients. The essence of these warnings is that marketing researchers have opportunities, but they have been too slow to take the initiative to seize and capitalize on these opportunities.

*I think you're called upon to do things if you prove you can make a contribution. You are what you make yourself. Shame on the people who just sit around and say,*

*"Nobody gives me any respect." Go out and get some respect. Go out and earn some respect.*

The proof that these opportunities exist comes from many of the sources identified by this research. The increase in demand is an affirmation of internal clients' belief in the value of marketing research. It is also a reflection of the times. Whether advocates of marketing research or not, internal clients cannot succeed without primary marketing research. There is simply too much uncertainty, too much competition, too much control in the hands of multiple customers, and too much at stake.

## NOTES

1. The authors acknowledge the contributions made by Edward Gray, Director of Marketing Research, SmithKline Beecham; Edward Leinbach, Manager of Marketing Research, SmithKline Beecham; William Carter, Manager of Marketing Research, SmithKline Beecham; Linda Kinzig, Manager of Marketing Research, SmithKline Beecham; Cynthia A. Ruiz, Senior Manager, Marketing Research, Rhone-Poulenc Rorer; David F. Cristoforo, Manager, Marketing Research, Rhone-Poulenc Rorer; Carl Kuebler, Manager of Marketing Research, Rhone-Poulenc Rorer; David Silverman, Director of Marketing Research and Decision Analysis, Sanofi Winthrop; Ken Slotnick, Associate Director of Marketing Research and Decision Analysis, Sanofi Winthrop; Julianna Simmons, Director of Marketing Research and Business Analysis, Boots Pharmaceuticals; Larry Belford, Executive Director, Marketing Information Services, CIBA-GEIGY; David Paddock, Director, Business Intelligence, Bock Pharmacal Company; Janet Reichmeier, Director, Business Information and Advertising, Marion Merrell Dow; Karen Abeyta, Account Executive, Walsh America/PMSI; and Ann Wasescha, Global Product Manager, 3-M Pharmaceuticals.

2. The term "consultants" is used here rather than the more common "suppliers" or "vendors" because there is ever-increasing demand for these individuals to deliver as consultants.

## REFERENCES

1. McNichol J. What senior management wants from marketing research. Med Market Media 1993;(May):38.

2. McNichol J. Senior management takes a closer look at marketing research. Med Market Media 1995;(Feb):38.

3. Julius M. Doing more with less in marketing research. Product Manage Today 1994;(Feb):25.

# Pharmaceutical Pricing
# at the Change of Millennia

## Mick Kolassa

The pricing of pharmaceuticals, like the pricing of many kinds of products, has traditionally been an uncertain endeavor. Regardless of the information gathered and the research and analysis conducted, one can never be sure that the price decided upon is the correct price. As we approach the millennium, may we expect this specter of uncertainty to remain? Will and Ariel Durant, noted historians of this century, advised: "If you want the present and the future to be different from the past, Spinoza tells us, find out the causes that made it what it was and bring different causes to bear." In business-specific terms, Drucker admonishes: "Long-range planning does not deal with future decisions, but with the future of present decisions." Let us review recent pharmaceutical pricing trends and decisions and consider the extent to which they may affect the future.

### *THE 1980s*

#### *Pricing Decisions*

Until very recently, few firms in the pharmaceutical industry committed adequate resources to pricing matters. Although this lack of formal attention to pricing is not unique to the pharmaceutical industry, the lack of a purposeful and coordinated approach to pricing within most firms has, to a

Mick Kolassa, M.B.A., is Senior Research Associate, Research Institute of Pharmaceutical Sciences, University of Mississippi, University, MS 38677.

[Haworth co-indexing entry note]: "Pharmaceutical Pricing at the Change of Millennia." Kolassa, Mick. Co-published simultaneously in *Journal of Pharmaceutical Marketing & Management* (Pharmaceutical Products Press, an imprint of The Haworth Press, Inc.) Vol. 10, No. 2/3, 1996, pp. 109-120; and: *Pharmaceutical Marketing in the 21st Century* (ed: Mickey C. Smith) Pharmaceutical Products Press, an imprint of The Haworth Press, Inc., 1996, pp. 109-120. Single or multiple copies of this article are available from The Haworth Document Delivery Service [1-800-342-9678, 9:00 a.m. - 5:00 p.m. (EST)].

great extent, brought about the pricing woes of the present. Pricing has been treated as an event, rather than a process, and each product has been priced in a different way, with pricing research and analysis approaches varying greatly from one product to the next.

Pricing functions and responsibilities were fragmented within most firms, with product managers and/or marketing research departments responsible for the bulk of analysis and consideration and top managers, relying on instinct, setting the list price for launch. Once commercialized, the price of the products tended to go in two directions, with list prices increasing at a fairly regular rate and contract prices, often managed by sales functions, continually moving downward in response to pressures (both real and imagined) in growing price-sensitive market segments.

These pricing activities tended to be performed in a discrete manner, with little or no coordination among the various parties and precious little coordination between the pricing strategy and the marketing plan for the products. Thus, it was not uncommon for marketing campaigns to tout a product's unique benefits and clinical value and point out the lack of appropriate alternatives while selling functions were busily discounting the same product to hospitals, nursing homes, and managed care groups, choosing to compete on price with older–even generic–agents.

These and other phenomena have interacted over the past 15 years to bring about the pricing environment currently faced by pharmaceutical makers. The use of generic drugs began to grow as a force in the early 1980s, and manufacturers of branded pharmaceuticals soon discovered that they could substantially raise the prices of their off-patent products without suffering severe losses in unit sales, beyond those already lost to generics, and thereby preserve sales levels as unit sales declined (1). This lack of price elasticity was due to two circumstances: the generally low prices for pharmaceuticals at the time and the traditional lack of price sensitivity by prescribing physicians (2). Manufacturers soon began to increase prices for patent protected products at nearly the same rate used for multisource drugs and, again, suffered no ill consequences, commercially. Simultaneously, they began to price new products at significant premiums over existing agents (3).

This rate of price growth, however, was noted by several public officials, including Senator David Pryor of Arkansas (4). Government hearings and investigations, together with attention by the media, brought great pressure on the American drug industry to change its pricing behavior.

It has long been accepted that new pharmaceutical products will enter the market at prices higher than those products preceding them to the market (5, 6). That both the pharmaceutical industry's chief critic, Senator Pryor, and the editor of the trade magazine serving the executives of that industry held the same conception of initial product pricing bears this out (7). Senator Pryor, in a 1990 *Health Affairs* article entitled "A Prescription for Higher Drug Prices," stated: "Rarely is a new product priced at a significantly lower level to attract market share from its competitors." John Curran, editor of *Pharmaceutical Executive,* noted the "new" pricing approach taken by Merck in the launch of Vasotec®, which was priced below its competitor, unlike other new agents (7). There appears to be a basic assumption among casual observers and critics alike that new agents will be priced higher than the older agents they are intended to replace in the market. But this trend has reversed itself.

A study by the Boston Consulting Group found that 21 of the 24 new chemical entities with direct competition that were introduced in the United States in 1991 and 1992 were priced, on average, 14% below the leading product in their class (8). For the most active chronic therapeutic areas, which include antihypertensives and other cardiovascular products, the discount averaged 36%. An investigation by researchers at the University of Mississippi found that only one product has been priced at a premium to direct competition since 1992 (3). This is a marked departure from the traditional and assumed pricing behavior of the past.

This change also leads us to challenge a general assumption about pharmaceutical prices–that generic products are less costly than brands. Grabowski and Vernon found that the prices for chemically equivalent generic versions of branded products varied in price by up to 50%, a finding that, according to economic theory, is not expected in a "commodity market" (9). Bloom and colleagues found that generic versions of branded pharmaceutical products were not always priced below the brand (10). In 66% of the products studied, the highest retail price found for generics was above the lowest price found for the brand of the same chemical makeup. While this study was based on a multipharmacy sample and there were no individual stores in which the price of the generic was higher than that of the competing brand, the distribution of retail prices was such that it could be concluded that generics are not always less costly than their branded counterparts.

Given that manufacturers have begun to set the prices of some of their newer products well below those of established brands and that it is the older, established brands that will receive generic competition because their patents will usually expire before those of their newer competitors, it is not unlikely that some new brands would be less costly than generic versions of some older competing products. This statement would seem to defy what might be considered common wisdom, but it can be demonstrated that some newer brands are, indeed, less costly than generic versions of their older competitors. A review of the National Prescription Audit and the pharmaceutical pricing database Price Check-PC reveals that the generic versions of nifedipine and diltiazem, two popular calcium channel blockers, at $1.17 and $1.47 per day, respectively, are priced above the newer branded calcium channel blockers DynaCirc® (isradipine, Sandoz, $1.04/day), Plendil® (felodipine, Astra-Merck, $0.92/day), and even an older brand, Calan SR® (verapamil, Searle, $1.16/day) (11, 12).

Even as the prices of newer agents have moderated the rate of price growth, the emergence of managed health care and hospital buying groups has brought about significant changes in the way in which pharmaceutical prices are determined. Aggressive bidding has caused a wide disparity between the retail prices and special contract prices of many pharmaceuticals (13). It appears to have become routine to offer discounts to specific customers.

The imposition of mandatory rebates based on discounts offered to other customers and paid to Medicaid programs, however, appears to have caused many firms to rethink their discount policies, as many have begun to increase prices to these segments (14, 15). Newly emerged pressure in the form of pharmacy and legislative accusations of discriminatory pricing has resulted in calls for "unitary pricing" to further narrow the discount gap.

Perhaps the most profound change in the pharmaceutical pricing environment in the 1980s was that the prescriber's choice of drug therapy came under the influence of payers and other intermediaries (16). Managed care, as opposed to traditional fee-for-service health insurance, grew from covering 5% of the insured population in the United States in 1980 to 80% of the insured population in 1991 (8). The growth of cost consciousness among payers appears to be a major force behind the change in the way manufacturers are setting their initial prices.

Finally, the useful life of pharmaceutical products has declined rapidly over the past 15 years. Early generic erosion and more direct competitors have brought about a shortened commercial life for a product, and lengthier times for approval have delayed the entry of many new products. As a result, the average pharmaceutical product has a "useful" life of approximately seven years (9). It is during this period of useful life that the product must generate sales and profits sufficient to finance the discovery and development of newer agents. Such a situation would appear to require higher than traditional prices if newer products are to be discovered.

Thus, the most recent trends in pharmaceutical pricing seem to be the combination of the moderation of price growth and the narrowing of discount ranges with increased need for price flexibility.

## The Expansion of Price Controls

Concurrent with the rise and fall of price growth in the United States, health care systems in other nations began to assert significant and growing control over pharmaceutical prices. Nations in northern Europe such as Germany, the Netherlands, and many Scandinavian nations, which began the decade of the 1980s with relatively free pricing for pharmaceuticals, began the decade of the 1990s with increasing restrictions (17). Contrasted with price growth in the U.S., which far exceeded the general rate of inflation during the 1980s, real prices for pharmaceuticals fell, relative to other goods and services, in most European nations (1). Even with this result–deflation of pharmaceutical prices-every European government has tightened controls over pharmaceutical prices in recent years.

It appears that government officials often confuse total spending with pricing problems, assuming that spending growth indicates excessive prices. Evaluation of European price control systems by the U.S. General Accounting Office has concluded that these programs are insufficient to control drug spending because, despite holding price growth below prevailing rates of inflation, total spending on pharmaceuticals continued to increase faster than the rate desired (18). Although such evaluations appear to ignore the inherent cost-effectiveness of pharmaceuticals and fail to consider the cost and quality consequences of the underutilization of prescription medications, these issues do not seem to affect decision making within government bodies (19).

A regulatory approach common to many nations is "reference pricing." Under such a system, the prices charged for a pharmaceutical product in several different nations are compared by a regulatory agency to assure that the prices charged in that nation are roughly equivalent to those charged in other nations. Canada, Portugal, and Italy now use such a system, and it appears likely that reference pricing will be adopted in the near future by Germany, the United Kingdom, and other nations.

The range of prices charged for the same product in different nations has been studied exhaustively, and it is often found that drug prices in the United States are higher than elsewhere (20, 21). Comparisons of international drug prices, often commissioned by the federal government, have brought about calls for a reference pricing system in the U.S. (21). A reference pricing system was prominently featured in the Clinton Health Plan of 1994. Although no such system is now in place, large disparities between prices in the U.S. and other nations will continue to be brought to the attention of regulators. A narrowing of international price "bands" appears to be in the works.

Many publicly financed health care provision systems were developed as government responses to the perceived problem of unmet medical need (22). While public officials in the United States often note the growth of Medicaid spending, especially for pharmaceuticals, and point to this growth as an indication of the need for tighter controls on health care costs, few have acknowledged the inevitability of cost increases in a system that provides goods and services free of charge (5, 23). As a former Minister of the British National Health Service noted, "There is virtually no limit to the amount of free medical care an individual is capable of absorbing."

Although the many programs provide a comprehensive package of health care goods and services and are meant to provide an overall benefit, the components of the benefit are often budgeted and managed as separate entities, resulting in conflicts between budgetary authorities (24). Many private insurers providing a pharmaceutical benefit operate the pharmacy program as a "carve out." This means that the pharmaceutical benefit is managed separately from the other aspects of the system. Thus, it has become common that the greater good of the total system is often subordinate to individual budget performance.

The budgetary problems of many government-provided health care programs are manifestations of a basic paradox in public transfer payment systems: as economic output and available tax revenues decrease, the demand for government assistance increases (22). Hence, as the demand for medical benefits–including pharmaceuticals–increases, the funds available to support those benefits are decreasing (25). Budgetary "crisis" in such a system is virtually guaranteed.

Over the past decade, studies have demonstrated that tight budgetary control of pharmaceuticals often results in increases in spending on other health care goods and services to offset any savings on drugs, a phenomenon known as the service substitution effect (26, 27). Other studies by Moore and Newman and Smith and Simmons have shown that the imposition of these controls does not even guarantee a reduction in spending on pharmaceuticals (28, 29). While some other studies in this area were questioned for their assumptions or methodologies, few studies have been produced that establish the ability of a restrictive formulary alone to save money in an outpatient setting (30).

Several cost control schemes, such as monthly prescription limitations and cost sharing, have also been shown to be less than optimal in controlling costs. As Nelson, Reeder, and Dickson found, restrictions or cost sharing can result in problems of underutilization, and underutilization can have a negative effect on health and result in cost increases (31). The imposition of a maximum number of prescriptions per beneficiary has been shown to have severe negative consequences, increasing total costs by increasing hospitalizations and nursing home admissions (32). Despite the preponderance of evidence that such restrictions are counterproductive, both in financial and health status terms, the bureaucratic faith in budgetary fragmentation appears unlikely to be shaken, and the continued micromanagement of the prescription budget can be expected in the future.

Thus, the key decision makers in prescription drug use appear to treat price in conflicting ways: physicians, in general, pay no attention to the price of a product, while other intermediaries can be said to consider little else. Price, then, plays very different roles in decision making, and firms must balance these opposing forces when setting prices.

## Pharmacoeconomics

In response to pricing pressures and to provide more information about their products, most pharmaceutical firms operating in the United States are, to some extent, engaged in pharmacoeconomic research. Although the field of pharmacoeconomic research is still in its relative infancy, there appears to be great hope that such studies will provide an appropriate basis for judging the economic value of pharmaceutical agents, as well as other health care interventions.

## THE FUTURE

The future environment that faces pharmaceutical manufacturers will be determined by the actions of customers, regulators, and the firms themselves. To expect significant changes in the decision-making and evaluative process of the governments is, perhaps, naive. It is thus incumbent upon the pharmaceutical firms and others to adapt to the decision-making styles of these officials.

The current trends that, if left unchallenged, are likely to continue include:

- Narrowing of the range of prices charged in different nations
- Further consolidation of buyers into more powerful groups
- More nonphysician decision makers
- Continued growth of generic drugs

- Continued increases in health care spending and scrutiny of drug budgets
- More attempts by pharmaceutical manufacturers to use price as a selling point
- Continued demands for discounts by many customers.

These combined–and often contradictory–trends will shape the pricing environment of the future. Many of the trends, several of which are troublesome for pharmaceutical makers, are self-imposed. Left unchecked or unchallenged, they will lead to a general lowering of price levels in the United States.

A seemingly ideal pricing environment would be one in which the value of pharmaceuticals is acknowledged and accepted and the prices are set according to the value of the product. Such an environment would clarify the "rules" for price determination and allow customers to evaluate the adoption of a new product. Pharmacoeconomic studies can facilitate such an environment if those sponsoring and performing such studies can agree on meaningful endpoints and health care administrators will admit that reductions in the pharmacy budget do not necessarily result in lower costs overall. The establishment of the economic value of a new pharmaceutical product would allow for a rational, transparent mechanism for the pricing decision, and we must continue to work for the acceptance of these studies. But three major factors, each emanating from regulatory bodies, stand in the way of value-based, rational pricing of pharmaceuticals. The first two factors are associated with price differentials among nations.

International price disparities will remain an issue of contention between those producing pharmaceuticals and those purchasing them. There are two distinct areas of concern: price differentials among developed nations and differences between the prices charged in developed versus undeveloped nations. The range of prices charged for the same medication in Europe can be quite broad. It is not uncommon that prices in France, Spain, and Greece are less than half the prices charged in Germany, the Scandinavian countries, or the United Kingdom. Such disparities will not be tolerated for long; thus, it is imperative that the price levels of pharmaceuticals in southern Europe be brought up to approach those in northern Europe and the United States. Failure to address this disparity will eventually lead to a downward adjustment of prices in the nations of northern Europe and North America.

As we look to emerging markets, on the other hand, price disparities will become a necessity. Regardless of the outcome of "price harmonization" in Europe, it must be admitted by producers and national authorities that citizens and governments of emerging nations cannot afford to pay the full value for many medical technologies. Part of the reason for this is that the current lack of health care technology in many nations implies the relatively low value, in economic terms, of health care interventions in general. Access to modern medicine, however, can help to free resources and to provide economic stimulation. But this cannot occur if emerging nations cannot afford to pay prices that are affordable in developed nations. For example, treatment for a disorder such as hepatitis is costly in developed nations, and a hepatitis cure could well be worth $1,000 or more per patient. But nations such as China, where the incidence of hepatitis is much greater than in the U.S. or Europe, may not be able to afford the $1,000 per patient because (1) that is far beyond what they now spend to treat the disorder and (2) national priorities are such that the funds that would be required to treat all appropriate patients could better be spent in other areas. In such cases, authorities in the developed countries must allow the product to be sold at its economic value ($1,000+) in their nations while it is being sold at a significantly lower price in China. Demands for price equity among all nations will deny needed medication to some nations and/or prevent drug manufacturers from earning the profits necessary to fuel the discovery and development of new agents.

The need to earn profits to fuel new drug discovery brings us to the last of the three factors: patent life. As periods of regulatory review and the time needed to comply with new government-imposed research requirements have lengthened, the effective patent life of a drug in the United States has become dangerously short. The trends toward lower prices at product launch and slower price growth, when combined with shortened periods of exclusivity, bring about the real danger that few new drugs will ever generate revenues sufficient to fund ongoing R&D. Clearly, new R&D efficiencies and/or initiatives that lengthen the period of exclusivity are necessary if drug discovery and development is to continue and research-based companies are to survive. A single year of extended exclusivity is worth approximately 18% of the average product's sales, or price. Each additional year of exclusivity, on average, generates as much profit as an average selling price that is 18% higher. Clearly, lower launch prices demand longer exclusivity.

## The Value of Pharmaceuticals

The main impediment to the appropriate and equitable pricing of pharmaceuticals lies in society's lack of acknowledgment of the value of pharmaceuticals, both in the macro sense–the financial savings gained through the use of pharmaceutical products as a whole–and from a micro perspective the–financial and patient-specific benefits from the appropriate use of many, if not most, new drugs. Part of the problem lies in the failure of society to take a systemwide view when evaluating health care, part in the long-term demonization of the pharmaceutical industry by critics, and a great deal in the industry itself.

The first two issues are self-explanatory; the third, and by far the most damaging, issue requires some discussion. Most pharmaceutical companies have actively worked in ways that devalue pharmaceutical products. The companies' own conduct has reduced the value of medications in the eyes of customers and society at large. For the past several years, prices in pharmaceutical markets have gone in two directions: increasing or holding firm in outpatient, cash-based markets and charging lower prices in hospital and managed care markets. Although these lower prices are in response to perceived market demands and are often accompanied by well-reasoned strategies for the discounts, public knowledge of these multitiered prices has brought many to question the appropriateness and equity of the non-discounted prices. Regardless of the legality of multiple price levels, which has been upheld time and again, two observations must be made:

1. There is little evidence that the deep discounting associated with managed care contracts has substantially affected the use of pharmaceutical products. In most therapeutic areas, the market share for individual products is the same in managed care markets as in cash markets.
2. The act of discounting, especially at some of the levels reported, signals (rightly or wrongly) that the company is willing to accept less for its product than it charges those who do not benefit from discounts. This is interpreted as overcharging.

Pharmaceutical firms must consider the financial and political consequences of pricing decisions and recognize that the granting of discounts is a pricing decision that cannot be made without careful consideration of the effect of those discounts on all aspects of the business. Firms must work to rationalize and manage all pricing activities while simultaneously working with public officials to recognize the value of pharmaceuticals as a cost control tool. I am afraid, however, that this value will not be acknowledged as long as perceptions of unfair pricing, brought on by wide price ranges, continue to exist.

# REFERENCES

1. Grabowski H, Vernon J. A sensitivity analysis of expected profitability of pharmaceutical research and development. Manage Dec Econ 1992;3(1):36-40.

2. Zelnio RN, Gagnon JP. The effects of price information on prescription drug product selection. Drug Intell Clin Pharm 1979;13:156-9.

3. Chukkapalli R, Kolassa EM, Ogilvey S, Hayman-Taylor T. The 15 year trend in prices at launch for outpatient prescription medications. Unpublished.

4. U.S. Senate. Special Committee on Aging. Prescription drug prices: are we getting our money's worth? Serial No. 101-F. Washington, DC, 1992.

5. Pryor D. A prescription for high drug prices. Health Aff 1990;9:101-9.

6. Dranove D. Medicaid drug formulary restrictions. J Law Econ 1989;23:143-62.

7. Curran JP. Strategic shifts in pricing policies. Pharm Exec 1986;6(Apr):92-4.

8. Boston Consulting Group. The changing environment for U.S. pharmaceuticals. New York: Boston Consulting Group, April 1993.

9. Grabowski HG, Vernon JM. Brand loyalty, entry, and price competition in pharmaceuticals after the 1984 Drug Act. J Law Econ 1992;23:331-50.

10. Bloom BS, Wierz DJ, Pauly MV. Cost and price of comparable branded and generic pharmaceuticals. JAMA 1986;256:2523-30.

11. IMS America. National Prescription Audit. October-December 1994. Plymouth Meeting, PA: IMS America.

12. Medispan Inc. Price Check-PC. December 1994. Indianapolis, IN: Medispan Inc.

13. Pathak DS, Klinger PA. Predictive factors in bid purchasing of antibiotics. Top Hosp Pharm Manage 1981;1(1):17-28.

14. Taylor S, Kucukarslan S, Sherrin T. Evidence and response to the impact of the Medicaid Drug Rebate Program (OBRA) on hospital pharmacy: a progress report from central Ohio. Hosp Pharm 1991;26:621-5.

15. Palumbo FB, Schondelmeyer SW, Miller DW, Speedie SM. Battered bottom lines: the impact of eroding pharmaceutical discounts on health-care institutions. Am J Hosp Pharm 1992;49:1177-85.

16. Wilensky GR, Blumberg LJ, Neumann PJ. Chapter 4. Pharmaceuticals and decision-making in the United States: cost consciousness and the changing locus of control. In: van Eimeren W, Horisberger B, eds. Socioeconomic evaluation of drug therapy. Berlin, New York: Springer-Verlag, 1988:32-45.

17. Wertheimer AI, Grumer SK. Overview of international pharmacy pricing. PharmacoEconomics 1992;2:449-55.

18. Anon. European price controls not sufficient to control drug spending without policies in place to control use. FDC Rep–Pinksheet 1994;(Jul 4):7-9.

19. Brown RE, Luce BR. The value of pharmaceuticals: a study of selected conditions to measure the contribution of pharmaceuticals to health status. Washington, DC: Battelle Medical Technology and Policy Research Center, March 1990.

20. Andersson F, McMenamin P. International price comparisons of pharmaceuticals–a review of methodological issues. London and Washington, DC: Battelle Medical Technology and Policy Centre (MEDTAP), 1992.

21. U.S. General Accounting Office. Prescription drugs: companies typically charge more in the United States than in Canada. Report to the Chairman, House Subcommittee on Health and the Environment, Committee on Energy and Commerce. GAO/HRD-920119. Washington, DC: September 1992.

22. Soumerai SB, Ross-Degnan D. Experience of state drug benefit programs. Health Aff 1990;9:36-54.

23. Goodman JC, Dolan EG. Economics of public policy. St. Paul, MN: West Publishing Company, 1985.

24. Kozma CM, Reeder CE, Lingle EW. Expanding Medicaid drug formulary coverage: effects on utilization of related services. Med Care 1990;28:963-76.

25. Reutzel TJ. The nature and consequences of policies intended to contain costs in outpatient drug insurance programs. Clin Ther 1993;15:752-64.

26. Bloom BS, Jacobs J. Cost effects of restricting cost-effective therapy. Med Care 1985;23:872-80.

27. Hefner DL. Cost effectiveness of a restrictive drug formulary. Washington, DC: National Pharmaceutical Council, 1980.

28. Moore WJ, Newman RJ. U.S. Medicaid drug formularies: do they work? PharmacoEconomics 1992;1(Suppl 1):28-31.

29. Smith MC, Simmons S. A study of the effects of formulary limitations in Medicaid programs. Admin Policy J 1982;2:169-98.

30. Rucker TD, Morse ML. The Medicaid drug program in Louisiana: critique of the Hefner-Pracon Study. Am J Hosp Pharm 1980;37:1350-3.

31. Nelson AA, Reeder CE, Dickson WM. The effect of a Medicaid drug co-payment program on the utilization of prescription services. Med Care 1984;22:724-36.

32. Soumerai SB, Avorn J, Ross-Degnan D, Gortmaker S. Payment restrictions for prescription drugs under Medicaid: effects on therapy, cost, and equity. N Engl J Med 1987;317:550-6.

# A Pharmaceutical Marketing Plan
## for the 21st Century:
## Sociopolitical Environment
## as a Marketing Factor

Francis B. Palumbo
Michael V. Laric

The sociopolitical environment is one of the uncontrollable business and marketing variables. This can be contrasted with controllable marketing variables (those over which the firm has control) such as product, price, place (distribution), and promotion (1). The firm decides which of several products it is going to develop, design, manufacture, or market. It then sets the price. In doing so, it must take into account a variety of factors, all of which are not under its control, such as the sociopolitical environment. The firm also decides where it will market. In determining its overall distribution, the firm must take into account its target markets. For a prescription drug, the target may be the primary practice physician, the health maintenance organization, or the pharmacy benefit management firm (PBM). Finally, depending on its product, the firm determines the promotional mix that it will use to promote its product. For prescription drugs, the most effective method of promotion in the past has been the

Francis B. Palumbo, Ph.D., is Associate Director of the Center on Drugs & Public Policy and Professor of Pharmacy Practice and Science at the University of Maryland School of Pharmacy, 20 North Pine Street, Baltimore, MD 21201. Michael V. Laric, Ph.D., is Associate Dean and Professor of Marketing at the Merrick School of Business, University of Baltimore.

[Haworth co-indexing entry note]: "A Pharmaceutical Marketing Plan for the 21st Century: Sociopolitical Environment as a Marketing Factor." Palumbo, Francis B., and Michael V. Laric. Co-published simultaneously in *Journal of Pharmaceutical Marketing & Management* (Pharmaceutical Products Press, an imprint of The Haworth Press, Inc.) Vol. 10, No. 2/3, 1996, pp. 121-130; and: *Pharmaceutical Marketing in the 21st Century* (ed: Mickey C. Smith) Pharmaceutical Products Press, an imprint of The Haworth Press, Inc., 1996, pp. 121-130. Single or multiple copies of this article are available from The Haworth Document Delivery Service [1-800-342-9678, 9:00 a.m. - 5:00 p.m. (EST)].

pharmaceutical marketing representative calling directly upon the prescriber. Other items in the promotional mix include general advertising, direct mail, and a variety of professional and continuing education programs.

Uncontrollable marketing variables, however, can be very serious constraints on the firm's ability to market. These include the economic environment, the social environment, the political environment, and the legal and regulatory environment. In this paper, we focus on the sociopolitical environment, and to the extent necessary, we also discuss the legal and regulatory environments. While in a classical marketing sense the company's business strategy is generally considered separately from the marketing strategy, in this paper, it is treated to the extent that the sociopolitical environment affects it. Finally, we discuss the sociopolitical environment as a marketing factor from a historical perspective beginning with the second half of the 20th century at about the time that the marketing concept evolved and was taking hold.

## THE 1960s: FROM STRICT SELF-RELIANCE
## TO PUBLIC ASSISTANCE

Beginning with the postwar era and through the 1960s, America viewed itself as a capitalistic nation where self-reliance was always a virtue. In the 1960s, a shift in the country's public policy focus began to develop, and vulnerable groups, principally the poor and the elderly, came to be viewed as deserving public help. In 1965 and 1966, Congress passed the Medicare and Medicaid acts, respectively. Medicare (Title XVIII of the Social Security Act) represents a health insurance program directed toward those 65 years of age and older. Prior to the passage of Medicare, the U.S. government had virtually no participation in taking care of the increasingly complex health care needs of the elderly population. This landmark legislation substantially helped to ease the health care burden of the elderly population. Medicare did not include a provision for outpatient drugs for the elderly population at the time.

Medicaid (Title XIX of the Social Security Act) is a program that provides health care for the poor. This program is administered through the states with funding from the federal government and includes outpatient drugs. From a pharmaceutical marketing perspective, attention was paid to the use of drugs by the Medicaid population and the marketing of drugs to physicians who treated Medicaid patients, while virtually no emphasis was placed on the outpatient drug needs of the Medicare population. Both Medicare and Medicaid have always covered drugs for inpatients, so this distinction was not focused upon to any extent by the pharmaceutical industry in marketing drugs to physicians for their hospitalized patients.

## THE 1970s: QUALITY AND THE BEGINNING OF MANAGED CARE

The quality of care became a major issue in the 1970s. Initially, the focus was on the inpatient environment for federally funded patients. The federal government established professional standards review organizations (PSROs) whose mission was to assure the quality and the economy of medical care (2-8). The prevailing wisdom was that if society was going to pay for much of the medical care provided to segments of citizens, then society could expect economical, high quality care for those recipient segments. The PSROs, later to become professional review organizations (PROs), concentrated primarily on the inpatient environment, including hospitals and long-term care facilities. Drugs, as part of the therapy in this environment, were included as part of the quality assurance effort. In that light, a number of efforts developed or matured that had an impact on pharmaceutical marketing.

Restrictive formularies known as hospital pharmacy and therapeutics committees (P&T committees) became much more active. With this increase in P&T Committee and formulary activity, pharmaceutical marketing was affected. There was a new focus on hospital pharmacists. Prior to this time, pharmaceutical marketing rarely focused on the pharmacist because the pharmacist did not exert influence on the selection of products. However, the pharmacist was and is a very influential member of the P&T Committee. The pharmacist's opinions on the inclusion (or exclusion) of drugs in the hospital formulary are given a great deal of respect. The main pharmaceutical marketing emphasis did not shift from the physician to the pharmacist but was essentially added to an already rigorous hospital marketing effort. Firms continued to focus on the hospital physicians. With this particular group, the stakes were perceived as very high because hospital physicians, especially those in training, establish prescribing patterns in the hospital that are then transferred to the community when that physician completes his or her residency. Later, some attention was focused on the community pharmacist as states began to repeal their antisubstitution laws. Now the pharmacist had some discretion over the dispensing of products in that he or she could substitute a generic drug for a brand-name drug. The pharmaceutical firms certainly could not control this change in the sociopolitical environment with regard to quality assurance, formularies, and repeal of antisubstitution laws, but they certainly were forced to take into account these sociopolitical changes as they developed and implemented their marketing plans.

During the same period of time, drug use review (DUR) was developed and began to mature as a method for assuring quality and economy of prescribing (9). While DUR focused on physician prescribing, pharmacist dispensing, and patient use of drugs, the lion's share of the attention was (and still is) on physician prescribing. DUR was virtually ignored by pharmaceutical marketers and many others for a number of years as being somewhat irrelevant to the drug selection process.[1]

As third-party drug programs evolved, much of the emphasis shifted to issues such as coverage and reimbursement. Now the pharmaceutical industry saw itself at risk and, once again, some uncontrollable sociopolitical variable was wielding its influence. The sociopolitical environment changed dramatically in 1973 when Congress passed the Health Maintenance Organization Act. This marks the beginning of managed care with a shift in emphasis to cost management. The act reflected the further change in societal attitudes from strict self-reliance through limited public assistance to, now, acceptance of greater government involvement. Such government involvement may have become politically feasible at this point primarily because of the shift in the sociopolitical environment and may be considered a continuation of the trend that lead to the passage of the Medicare and Medicaid acts.

## THE 1980s: THE DECADE OF HIGHER PRICES AND DRGs

During the 1980s, pricing and product development dramatically changed the face of pharmaceutical marketing. The controllable variable of price dramatically escalated. In fact, medical care expenditures, in general, increased at a rate that far exceeded the consumer price index for all goods.

These price increases gave rise to a change in the emphasis from quality assurance to cost management. While quality assurance efforts matured and expanded, they represent only part of the overall environment. The payment mechanism for inpatient care was reorganized with the advent of diagnosis related groups (DRGs) (10). As with other initial efforts, these focused on the inpatient setting for federally funded patients. DRGs represent a direct effort to place some limits on hospital costs and to introduce into the mix the idea of risk sharing. Pharmacy changed, to a certain extent, as a result of DRGs. Hospital pharmacy now became a cost center rather than a revenue center. The hospital pharmacist is now often faced with a variety of choices regarding services and products within a fixed overall budget. Thus there is a heightened emphasis on marketing to the hospital pharmacist, and this will undoubtedly continue into the 21st century.

However, the hospital pharmacist is not the only pharmaceutical health professional who exerts influence over the market through such variables as restrictive formularies. The managed care pharmacist covers many tasks, including drug use review, restrictive formularies, and reimbursement. Many of these pharmacists are associated with pharmacy benefit management companies (PBMs). At the moment, PBMs influence a great deal of the pharmaceutical market and are the focus of pharmaceutical marketing efforts now and into the 21st century.

## THE 1990s: THE DAWN OF A NEW ERA

With the appearance of managed care in the 1980s, the stage was set for its profound impact on pharmaceutical marketing toward the end of the 20th century. Managed care, in one form or another, will continue to dominate pharmaceutical marketing well into the 21st century. To accept this statement, one has only to consider the Omnibus Budget Reconciliation Act of 1990 (OBRA 90) (11). Under OBRA 90, pharmaceutical manufacturers are required to provide rebates to state Medicaid programs, and these rebates are in relation to the amount of a company's product that has been dispensed to Medicaid recipients within a state.

While OBRA 90 is directed toward Medicaid programs, the idea of rebates has expanded into the private sector and into other areas of the public sector. PBMs, for example, negotiate rebates on behalf of their clients. With Medicaid and private rebate programs, we have seen the pharmaceutical marketing emphasis shift from product competition to price competition. This trend will undoubtedly continue for the near term; however, when rebates have been literally exhausted, other pharmaceutical marketing strategies will be in order. One of these is pharmacoeconomics, which includes outcomes research (12). Pharmaceutical manufacturers once marketed heavily based on the distinction between their product and another company's product to treat a similar disease state with differential effectiveness. After OBRA 90, this evolved into a price competitive market. But in the future, pharmaceutical manufacturers are expected to distinguish their products from other companies' products on the basis of superior cost-effectiveness, utility, or patient outcomes. To remain competitive, pharmaceutical companies have applied these pharmacoeconomics methods to existing products to distinguish them from other manufacturers' products. However, the trend now and into the future is for manufacturers to include pharmacoeconomics as an integral part of drug development. This is particularly important because part of the emphasis of drug development has moved to biotechnology.

Despite failed federal health care reform efforts in recent years, substantial sociopolitical forces have had an impact on the structure of the health care system, and they can have a profound impact on pharmaceutical marketing. One particular change is probably more one of attitude than of substance and relates to the federal government's efforts to promote legislation on health care reform. Under the present administration, much of the emphasis has been on access to care, but not at the expense of ignoring cost and quality issues.

Had the Health Security Bill passed, it could have created a new structure for delivering health care to virtually everyone in the U.S. It did contain provisions for inclusion of prescription drugs, but it also changed the major focus of health care delivery in this country toward a managed care, or managed competition, model. Such a change certainly would have had a profound impact on the marketing of pharmaceuticals in that a much larger percentage of the population would now be in a managed care environment and the pharmaceutical companies would have to face these new marketing issues with regard to a larger share of their products. Other issues that will occupy our sociopolitical environment include the marriage of genetic engineering to pharmaceutical drug developments, the emergence of new dispensing technologies, and globalization.

## BACK TO THE FUTURE: SOCIOPOLITICAL ISSUES AND MARKETING OPPORTUNITIES

Biotechnology has emerged as a major force in health care, and it is associated with major sociopolitical issues. For example, social and ethical issues abound with regard to genetically engineered drugs, patents on live beings, and the ethical issues involved with these developments. What potential effects will the products have on the environment? How does science deal with emergent life forms? Do we have the right or obligation as a society to regulate this branch of science? When we consider gene therapy, are we entering into areas the consequences of which we do not fully understand? These are just a few of the questions with which we must deal as the scientific community and the pharmaceutical industry continue to work and market in the biotechnology field.

There are also legal and political issues involved with genetically engineered drugs. For example, patent issues have arisen with regard to similarly engineered genetic drugs that might differ because of some minor deviation, such as an extra amino acid. In addition, there has been a fair amount of controversy over the effect of genetically engineered drugs on the operation of the Orphan Drug Act. The sociopolitical environment was a major influence in Congress's passage of the Orphan Drug Act, an act providing incentives to pharmaceutical companies to develop drugs for groups of less than 200,000 affected patients where the development of that drug might otherwise be unprofitable. Major brand-name companies may lose money on an orphan drug but see it as part of their social responsibility. However, small biotechnology companies may need the proceeds to survive, so they must charge inordinately high prices for these products. Occasionally, the interests of these biotech companies and those of more traditional pharmaceutical manufacturers conflict.

Sociopolitical trends affect social choices which can, in turn, influence the development of therapies or treatments and at the same time affect government policies. Generally, a drug must go through three phases of clinical trials under an investigational new drug application (INDA) before it can be approved for marketing. These phases are both time-consuming and expensive. The emergence of acquired immunodeficiency syndrome has somewhat changed the prevailing attitude about this. AIDS is a disease that threatens the very fiber of society and certainly has had an impact on the sociopolitical environment and the development of drugs. Activists/advocacy groups dramatically increased their activities and put pressure on the government to speed up the process of drug development. In response to this, the FDA stopped AZT trials after Phase II and approved the drug because the results appeared so dramatic. Afterward, the agency promulgated new regulations which included both the treatment IND regulations and the accelerated approval regulations (13, 14). The treatment IND allows for access to experimental drugs for the purpose of treatment in patients with serious or life-threatening illness. Accelerated approval regulations, on the other hand, allow for faster marketing approval time for drugs to treat serious or life-threatening illness. These accelerated approval regulations actually give the FDA some control over the prescribing and/or dispensing process. Regulations such as these probably affect the initial decision to develop and then market a drug more than the marketing strategy after the drug is developed. Suffice it to say that regulations such as these will be a major factor well into the 21st century, and the pharmaceutical industry will need to consider these when deciding which products to pursue and to market.

In our present sociopolitical environment, there is still a great deal of pressure to control costs. With all of these changes, the pharmaceutical industry is focusing its attention on how it might change its marketing philosophy and activities. One way in which the pharmaceutical industry has reacted in a somewhat revolutionary manner is the tendency toward vertical integration. This is a direct result of changes in the health care system associated with the sociopolitical environment. While some pharmaceutical manufacturers are purchasing PBMs to try to maintain market share, the sociopolitical environment once again comes into play in that societal interests must be balanced. Society wants decreased costs and continued access to health care, but society also wishes to be free from artificial market constraints and antitrust violations.

Companies are also entering the arena of disease management. Disease management is defined differently depending on whom one might ask at any particular point in time. However, as some would envision it, pharmaceutical manufacturers will actually enter into capitation agreements with managed care organizations whereby the manufacturers will agree to accept the risk for managing the disease (drug therapy) of patients in that managed care organization. As an example, the manufacturer may have a line of products dealing with hypertension and will capitate all of the hypertensive patients for antihypertensive therapy. To do this, however, the manufacturer will probably need to have access to a broad range of products within a broad therapeutic class (for example, antihypertensives). This may be accomplished through horizontal integration. Companies will merge and expand their product lines. Such expansion could include purchase or startup of generic manufacturing operations so that they can actually provide all or most of the products for which they are attempting to capitate the benefit. This type of activity is only in the neophyte stage now, but it is something that will surely continue into the 21st century.

Integration and alliances will continue as global markets develop. The world pharmaceutical market has certainly shrunk, especially after the establishment of the European Community (EC). Globalization enhances the ability to buy companies from other countries. For example, Squibb and Novo began to market insulin in the United States. Squibb had the distribution system and Novo had the insulin. Ultimately, pursuant to an agreement between the two companies, Novo took over the entire insulin production and distribution system. Strong companies often form alliances to produce a particular product. As an example, Siemens and Corning joined together to produce optic fiber, a product which neither could produce on its own. Scientific collaboration is made much easier in a global market through increased communications and use of cyberspace. Scientists have been collaborating internationally for generations. Yet, in this new global economy, collaboration is extending to regulatory and marketing efforts.

With enhanced communications, special interest consumer groups can now have a tremendous effect on the marketing of pharmaceuticals. As an example, special interest groups of consumers with certain illnesses communicate routinely through the Internet and share information on treatments for their illnesses, especially drug treatments. While consumerism may differ from country to country and society to society, the world population is certainly growing older. This fact, coupled with socialized medicine in many countries, can represent countless opportunities for joint ventures. Joint ventures can take the form of manufacturing alliances, quality assurance efforts such as DUR or formulary development, and innovative marketing efforts.

In this paper, we have attempted to detail a number of the issues related to the sociopolitical environment as a marketing factor for pharmaceuticals in the 21st century. Pharmaceutical marketing plans must take into account shorter life cycles for products. This is a direct result of changes in the health care marketplace which would include managed care, therapeutic substitution, and prior authorization programs. This also relates to pricing, which will become more visible as third parties tighten financial controls and capitalize on managed care principles. Competition from biotechnology upstart firms will increase, bringing to the marketplace new and exciting products and techniques that compete with more traditional pharmaceuticals. The global marketplace will continue to grow, and standards such as those being developed in the EC will make marketing and advertising much more predictable. Managed health care will continue to change as the health care system is reformed, whether through federal or state efforts. Large buyers will extract special prices through negotiations, and marketing directed toward physicians will change as physicians continue to become less of a decision-making force in the pharmaceutical marketplace.

In many respects, sociopolitical factors will continue to some of the most important, if not *the* most important, variables affecting the marketing of pharmaceuticals in the 21st century. As the sociopolitical environment changes, approaches to access, financing, and marketing of health care will also change.

## NOTES

1. DUR was seen as an activity that was important yet outside the scope of marketing decisions. Not until much later, perhaps with the passage of the Medicare Catastrophic Coverage Act of 1988, did the pharmaceutical industry finally recognize DUR as a force to be reckoned with.

# REFERENCES

1. McCarthy EJ. Basic marketing: a managerial approach. Homewood, IL: Richard D. Irwin, Inc., 1971.

2. Hess AE. A ten-year perspective on Medicare. Public Health Rep 1976;91:299-302.

3. Weikel MK. A decade of Medicaid. Public Health Rep 1976;91:303-8.

4. Davis K. Achievements and problems of Medicaid. Public Health Rep 1976;91:309-16.

5. Saward EW. Medicare, medical practice, and the medical profession. Public Health Rep 1976;91:317-21.

6. Donabedian A. Effects of Medicare and Medicaid on access to and quality of health care. Public Health Rep 1976;91:322-31.

7. McLachlan G. A foreign view of the United States under Medicaid and Medicare. Public Health Rep 1976;91:332-5.

8. McNerney WJ. Health insurance in the Medicare years. Public Health Rep 1976;91:336-42.

9. Knapp DA, Knapp DE, Brandon BM. Drug use review: a manual system. J Am Pharm Assoc 1973;NS13:417-21.

10. Williams SJ, Torrens PR. Introduction to health services. 2nd ed. New York: John Wiley and Sons, 1984.

11. Brushwood D, Catizone C, Coster J. OBRA 90: what it means to your practice. US Pharm 1992;(Oct):64-74.

12. Bootman JL, Townsend RJ, McGhan WF. Principles of pharmacoeconomics. Cincinnati: Harvey Whitney Books Company, 1991.

13. 21 C.F.R. Section 312.34 et seq.

14. 21 C.F.R. Section 314.500 et seq.

# Retail Pharmacists as a Marketing Target

## Michael J. O'Neill

*It is a paradox that in our time of drastic rapid change when the future is in our midst devouring the present before our eyes, we have never been less certain about what is ahead of us.*
— Eric Hoffer

### INTRODUCTION

In any discussion of the needs of the retail pharmacist in the 21st century, we first need to develop a concept of how this segment of pharmacy will be functioning at that time. To construct such a vision of the future, I will take cues from existing models for some significant elements affecting pharmacy: patient, payer, manufacturer, and prescriber. I will then attempt to imagine how these elements might change as a result of the external and internal forces operating on them. By taking a best guess of the strength of these forces as applied against these current models, I hope to develop a direction in which the model is heading. Using this direction, we can develop a concept of how retail pharmacy will itself respond to the evolved models. By no means am I suggesting that I possess the prescience to construct a detailed, accurate forecast of the future. At most, I think that this paper will provide an indication of the direction that pharmacy will take. At the least, I hope it will be the basis for a concept that readers can integrate into their own personal views about the future.

---

Michael J. O'Neill is Vice President for Professional Operations at Revco D.S., Inc., 1925 Enterprise Parkway, Twinsburg, OH 44087.

[Haworth co-indexing entry note]: "Retail Pharmacists as a Marketing Target." O'Neill, Michael J. Co-published simultaneously in *Journal of Pharmaceutical Marketing & Management* (Pharmaceutical Products Press, an imprint of The Haworth Press, Inc.) Vol. 10, No. 2/3, 1996, pp. 131-148; and: *Pharmaceutical Marketing in the 21st Century* (ed: Mickey C. Smith) Pharmaceutical Products Press, an imprint of The Haworth Press, Inc., 1996, pp. 131-148. Single or multiple copies of this article are available from The Haworth Document Delivery Service [1-800-342-9678, 9:00 a.m. - 5:00 p.m. (EST)].

## THE PATIENT

A simplified description of the traditional patient is that of an individual who seeks medical attention when he or she experiences discomfort, distress, or signs of disease. For the most part, this patient has been free to see the physician of his or her choice and has taken responsibility for payment, even if payment was administered through an insurer or other third party to the transaction. This patient places himself or herself in the hands of the system and generally does not take ownership for compliance with medical or good health practices. The patient tends to treat his or her body like an instrument of utility that when damaged is simply entered into the health care system for repair.

Recent changes in the management of health care are converting this patient into an individual who is more and more expected to maintain health and prevent sickness. The new system is also directing the patient to a restricted list of health care providers. The selection of these providers is based principally on the criteria of economics. The patient becomes "registered" in a health plan and is expected to follow the rules and protocols of that plan.

I believe the development of this model will continue in its current direction of patient control. The forces acting on it are financial, are mainly external, and are enormously potent. Most individuals cannot accept the financial risk for the staggering amounts of money that might be required for their health care and so seek group protection, usually through some form of insurance. In doing so, they share their risk with other members of the group but forfeit most of their rights to health care selection. The "group protector" is in control of the patient and often in control of who it will and will not protect.

The essence of this model–registration and control–will only be intensified as technology makes control of individuals easier. In the future, all of us will have a portable *medical* identification, new generations being assigned at the fetal stage. This is not the same as an insurance card. The identification I am referring to will record our health changes and status from birth until death. The culmination of the mapping of the human genome will allow the analysis of DNA samples to predict our susceptibility to hereditary disease as well as our relative strengths in various organs of the body. This identification will link us with other members of our family tree whose health will be subject to the same analyses.

The data collected through this mechanism will be enormously valuable for several reasons. Researchers will have a vast pool of demographics and population variances from which to draw information. Statisticians will be able to assign individuals to risk pools for targeted health care and preventive activities early in a life cycle. Allocation for resources against disease will be more accurate, and even Social Security will find use for this data through enhancement of the actuarial design of benefits, which will be distributed based more on need than on earnings.

This identification will be electronically encoded, starting with something as simple as a bar code that has only the simple purpose of enrolling an individual in a health data bank. Eventually, it will be much like a computer disk that will maintain files of information. To illustrate how close we are to such a system, consider this excerpt from an invitation to attend the Eleventh International Symposium on the Creation of Electronic Health Record Systems and Global Conference on Patient Cards. The symposium was held March 14-19, 1995, and was sponsored by the Medical Records Institute. This group was formed in 1981 to work for the advancement in implementation of electronic medical records.

Tutorial 27
Clinical Use of Patient Cards

Patient cards equipped with some form of memory must be designed to allow free, easy flow of information from the card to the care providers' systems, and they must be able to accept information from care providers as well. Criteria for such a bi-directional data transfer capability would include well-planned compatibility between the cards and the care givers' systems, and easy encoding/decoding of the narrative clinical text, in order to protect the patient's right to privacy, and to prevent any alteration of the clinical data. This tutorial will discuss the various aspects of the problems in a clinical settings [sic], and demonstrations will be given involving several vendors' cards to show the technical feasibility of controlling in a large system the compatibility, confidentiality and data integrity problems.

The most significant words in this paragraph are "demonstrations will be given." This is not the future; this is now.

For privacy protection, the level of access to the information will vary according to the provider. A laboratory technician, for example, might have access to previous lab values but not family history or other medical information. An emergency medical technician might only have access to current disease states, drug treatment, and personal emergency contact numbers. An admitting hospital will be able to access all medical and financial information. Additionally, unauthorized printing or retrieval of certain data from an individual's card will activate a method to disable the system that is attempting it.

This card will become our single most important piece of identification. It will follow us through childhood (think immunizations, childhood diseases), the military (think geographic stations, wounds), career (think exposure to environment, on-the-job injuries), retirement (think surgery, chemical interventions), and death (think legacy of data).

It will be necessary to present the card for any health care. There will be a ubiquitous ability to update all health events, the update being automatically put into the proper access file. Because all transactions will be electronically linked with data banks, fraud and abuse of the medical system will become more difficult.

The very act of involving patients in such a controlled environment will continue the recent trend toward emphasizing the individual's responsibility for his or her own health care. Much like today when a child is born with a health deficiency and parents are instructed in how to deal with it, parents will be given predictive information about health risks for their newborn–even if born "healthy"–and will be able to respond with appropriate nutritional, physical, and psychological support. The same will apply to themselves.

## *THE PAYER*

We have several current models for payers of health care. These include various types of insurance programs, the government, employers, and individuals. They are all driven by a common need to control costs. Indeed, for many providers who deal with payers, cost often seems to be payers' primary goal, moving patient care to a subordinate position. *Managed care* becomes equated with *managed costs*.

Excluding the individual, payers predominantly attempt cost control through various contracting arrangements with providers who deliver the services their populations require. These arrangements typically go beyond pricing to include hours of availability, transaction media, systems compatibility, generic substitution rates, interventions on behalf of the payer, etc. Some of these requirements have conflicting goals for pharmacists. For example, a payer wants a pharmacist to contact a physician to switch a brand-name prescription to a generic at the same time that it wants a member "wait time" penalty imposed. Economic survival aside, a provider's main task is rapidly becoming accommodation of all of the different payers' rule sets and systems requirements.

This model is under pressure from both internal and external sources. Internally, payers are under constant competitive pressure to hold down costs. They attempt this by containing the delivery and selection of procedures/products as well as bargaining for reduced payments for the same, as previously described. Externally, the source of the pressure varies more by type of payer. The insurance model is under pressure from competition, the government, its own members, the employers who reimburse it for its services, and the providers who are being forced to "take it or leave it." In my judgment, the greatest pressure on this model is coming from the government. It appears that the insurers feel that way also, as demonstrated by the amount of money spent by the Health Insurance Association of America (remember the "Harry and Louise" ads?) to defeat legislative health reform.

The government payer model is under external pressure from virtually the same list, including competition. Ironically, even government is putting performance pressure on government. Witness states bailing out of federal programs to form their own health care entities. Twenty-four states now have HCFA waivers.

Strong social pressures are also at work. In the past, the wealthy could afford health care and the very poor could not. Health care was divided by social status. The "Great Society" of the 1960s conferred a health entitlement on the poor, raising the level of their care. Spiraling health costs were simultaneously at work on the upper classes, slowly reducing the level of their care. As the system began to price services based on community comparisons through mechanisms such as diagnostic related groups (DRGs), the two levels of health care started to move to eliminate the difference between the classes. Like it or not, the care that one receives is being gradually reduced to the lowest common denominator. One could project that there will come a time when all care–at least through a contracted payer–will be identical.

I believe the net effect of these economic and social forces is that payers of the future will consolidate to a very few in number. This may occur through the formation of regional health care purchasing alliances, as proposed during the recent health legislation efforts. We may even see a single payer, the government. Dealing with a small number of payers will provide some basis for standardization of benefits and systems requirements. Health providers will have only a few contractors to satisfy and can eventually return their energies to patient care.

The current payer methodology of achieving cost savings by simply mandating lower provider reimbursement is obviously self-limiting. There will come a time in the search for what payers call "low cost provider" when there are no more costs that can be removed. Payers will gradually place more emphasis on control of services and procedures. They will be assisted in part by the patient identification discussed earlier. Step therapies, disease management protocols, diagnostic procedures, etc. will all be spelled out for individual patient treatment. Any costs incurred outside of these parameters may be paid for by the individual or perhaps by the payer after an arbitration process has validated the success of the procedure. Continuity of care will be insured. Patients will be enrolled with a limited number of payers who will be able to track the patients' activities, intervene when appropriate, and even apply penalties against patients who refuse to comply.

The true cost of prescription drugs is one large remaining expense from which payers will be able to extract reductions. Payers for prescription drugs will eventually force the abandonment of rebates from the manufacturers. Rebates will be replaced with negotiated prices for products. The payer will purchase products *directly* from the manufacturers, not as in the current system of *indirectly* from the manufacturers through the providers (pharmacies).

I believe this will occur for several reasons. The first is that the current system of rebates does not make sense. It is something that the industry backed into as a solution for manufacturers who needed their products included in controlled formularies and as a partial offset for class of trade pricing. Medicaid was among the first to recognize the differences in product pricing from manufacturers and forced the issue. Simply explained, manufacturers under OBRA 90 were required to return to the government a calculated difference between their best price and the average manufacturer's price to wholesalers. Rebates received under this mandate in 1992 by the states totaled approximately $1.1 billion.

We would be hard pressed to explain by logical means how the drug rebate system came about. Consider that a payer is agreeing to buy the drug from a pharmacy which bought the drug from a manufacturer which returns part of this purchase price back to the payer. In addition, consider that the payer who buys the drug from the pharmacy is attempting to control costs, not by reducing the true cost from the manufacturer, but by constantly lowering the difference between the price *that the manufacturer sets* for the pharmacy and what the payer wants to pay for the dispensing. It would seem that the average car buyer understands the shell game of rebates better than the payer segment of the health care industry.

Another reason that I don't believe the rebate system will continue is that, by and large, the rebate is being collected and distributed, sometimes negotiated, by an entity called a pharmacy benefit manager (PBM). For this service, the PBM keeps part of the rebate. The other purposes of the PBM are to register patients within a plan and to control the medication benefits distributed to plan members. The PBM's position seems to be that of a classic middleman and probably won't exist in the future, its role being negated by the direct managed care activities of the payers.

Yet another reason for this direct purchase approach is that the manufacturers have their own economic, marketing, and distribution needs that this scenario would meet.

## THE MANUFACTURER

The current model for manufacturers is a familiar one, and I will only cover the points affected by the model. Manufacturers fall into two groups: an innovator, brand-name group and a multisource, generic group. The innovator engages in research and new drug development. The drug is introduced through a marketing network and distributed either directly or through wholesalers. The generic group relies on copying successful, highly accepted drugs after they come off patent protection. Recently, there has been a great deal of consolidation among manufacturers, and this trend will undoubtedly continue. There are predictions that eventually all high-volume products will come from approximately ten manufacturers. Taking positions in the new health care environment, manufacturers have concluded recent acquisitions of wholesalers, mail-order pharmacies, and pharmacy benefit managers.

Pressure on this model is both internal and external. For survival, a manufacturer must have a needed product, significant market share, and distribution capabilities. Capital investment in research, development, and marketing is enormous. Manufacturers are under extreme regulatory control and constant price pressures. They are in an industry that produces increasingly expensive, inelastic goods and that seems to be forever flirting with the threat of government price control.

As stated before, I believe that, in the future, manufacturers will abandon the rebate process and simply price their drugs directly to the ultimate payer. This scenario will come about as a result of some of the changes already discussed. There will be a limited number of payers who will control large groups of people. Drug use within a payer population will be easily predictable based on data from the patient identification system. As we have discussed, this identification goes beyond the role of data collection currently being performed by a PBM. It will identify health conditions which will be linked to corresponding therapies as controlled by the payer. Patient demographics provided to a payer will locate individual patients within a given radius of provider pharmacies in a network. The payer will know which drugs (formulary) these pharmacies will need, but as we will see, perhaps not all pharmacies will be allowed to dispense all medications.

When a pharmacy is accepted into the network, it will receive its drug supply from the manufacturer. The drugs will be in unit of use packaging, the size of the package dictated by the established therapy parameters and whether the drug is newly prescribed or a maintenance refill. Newly prescribed drugs may be dispensed as starter packages.

Each package will have a specific bar code so that the manufacturer will know which pharmacy has the inventory, and through participation in the electronic information system, when it was dispensed. Patient days supply will be captured via the payer so that both manufacturer and payer will know when the next dispensing will occur, and there will be automatic replenishment. The bar code will assist in recalls, both for out-of-date items and regulatory reasons. In fact, there should be no out-of-date items to return. The manufacturer will have the opportunity to move inventory between pharmacies based on movement within the network, and it will have predictive data to match production with usage. All of these elements will decrease manufacturing costs.

What other kind of cost savings would a manufacturer gain under this scenario? First, it would negate the need for a sales force and would limit marketing efforts. Drugs would be judged on a medical value to cost ratio, the data for which would come from measuring outcomes. The information for success or failure of drug therapy will be found in that rich resource of patients within a network who are being tracked on their health identification card. Second, the manufacturer could now accurately predict expenses for distribution for all products, including the expense associated with new products entry. No longer would the manufacturer have to arrange to put an item in every retailer or every wholesaler while having little or no control over how many of the items or which ones are being inventoried. Products would only go to network pharmacies in appropriate quantities. Third, consider the dilemma faced with the introduction of vastly more expensive biotech products, which are predicted to be the wave of the future. Distributing them only to a limited number of providers will be an economic necessity. In fact, we have a model for this now with the Betaseron® program. Fourth, as stated, it would virtually eliminate the need for a returned goods policy. Fifth, because the price is direct between payer and manufacturer, the difficult issues of pricing tiers among classes of trade and having to maintain rebate records are resolved.

The advantage of direct purchasing for payers is that they are now truly controlling the prices of the drugs for their members. There would be very little doubt about costs, allowing accurate plan design that would benefit the payer, the patient, and the provider. Accurate data to forecast costs would allow payer and manufacturer to work together to develop low risk, participatory capitation programs that are mutually beneficial.

## THE PRACTITIONER

Much has been written about future changes in health care that will affect the practice of medicine. Most of the predictions discuss increased emphasis on the role of a primary care physician who will act as a gate-keeper, controlling patient access to "necessary" specialized treatment. Physicians acknowledge an increasingly controlled health care environment and
reliance on computer systems that will guide practice standards. Like other providers in the health care system, physicians are experiencing pressure to change that is mainly external and economic. I will only address the role of the practitioner as it relates to prescribing.

Physicians will continue to leave private practice and migrate toward group practice. This movement will be accelerated by the vertical integration of hospitals and clinics and by enrollment in Community Health Information Networks (CHINs). These networks fit the previous scenarios of patient identification and payer control. In fact, they are most likely to be the precursor of regional health alliances.

CHINs, although limited in existence, are already a fact of life. Many more are in the planning stages. The problems previously discussed in dealing with a large number of payers are much more evident in the fledgling struggles of CHINs. They are not standardized in their control, systems requirements, procedures, confidentiality protocols, etc. However, we can safely predict that efforts like those of the Medical Records Institute will bring standardization. Like payers, the standardization will come, lowering barriers to consolidation, encouraging their evolution into some few in number.

A physician will be linked to all community health care activities via a CHIN. Portable, hand-held radio frequency devices will allow them connection without being tied to a fixed terminal. They will be able to order lab tests, get results, receive an update on a patient in a hospital, prescribe medications, have access to medical literature, and collaborate with colleagues, all within an electronic network. The ultimate effect will be an overwhelming demand on their time. Combined with the continuing emphasis on primary care, more and more of the current physician's duties will be taken over by other health care professionals. The model for this is the nurse practitioner or physician assistant. More than likely, this position will evolve into a new health professional who will be some hybrid of physician assistant with limited prescribing authority.

At present, there are several computer systems that link physicians to pharmacies. Their current use is for authorization of refills or issuing new prescriptions. Their main advantage, according to one PBM, is that they will help the physician prescribe drugs that are in the formulary and perform all of the necessary DUR functions before the prescription is transmitted to the pharmacy. Amazingly, PBMs claim that participation in this system by a pharmacy will enhance the role of the pharmacist and prove his or her professional value, thereby providing the PBM the rationale to increase pharmacist reimbursement. It seems that the opposite would be more likely. The system as proposed is merely transferring the traditional role of the pharmacist to the physician's office, hardly a reason to increase the pharmacist's reimbursement. At any rate, the use of electronic prescribing in some form or fashion seems to be in our future.

## THE RETAIL PHARMACY

We are all familiar with the model for retail pharmacy. Pharmacies are staffed mainly by graduates of a baccalaureate degree program and can be located in virtually any setting–as free-standing, in clinics, in grocery stores, as chain drugstores, within mass merchandisers, etc. Retail pharmacies represent the health care resource most accessible to the public. They process prescriptions on demand without appointment. They consult with the public on a variety of minor ailments, and most inventory and sell over-the-counter remedies. Most participate in multiple prescription provider networks. Inventory for any drug, in any location, is virtually assured. Various types of practice can be found in retail pharmacy, including long-term care, IV infusion, and compounding. We will consider only the model that deals with the general practice of providing ambulatory care prescription services.

There are both internal and external forces acting on pharmacy. Generally speaking, internal pressures come from the need for economic survival, professional associations, regulatory boards, and educational requirements, while external pressures come from payers, regulatory agencies, and competition. Given these pressures and considering that there is some validity in the preceding outline of future health care, we can forecast that retail pharmacy will evolve along the following lines.

A patient will still receive a prescription at a pharmacy. All prescriptions will be transmitted electronically within a health network. For simplicity, we will assume that network is a CHIN, but it could be part of a regional or government health alliance (payer). The transmission process of a prescription will not represent fulfillment. The CHIN will simply hold this information until the prescription is delivered to the patient. If delivery is not validated, there will be a protocol in place for compliance intervention and the pharmacy will be prompted to contact the patient. Much like today's override facility for prescription interventions, the pharmacist will reply to the CHIN as to the reasons the patient did not accept the medication. The CHIN will have its own set of procedures to ensure patient compliance. The logic used here is that there was payment rendered for an examination or other procedure that resulted in the issuance of a necessary prescription. The patient will be held responsible for taking the medicine or for payment of the service.

The patient's identification card, which handles his or her health record, will not be updated until the prescription is delivered to the patient. Delivery will simultaneously update the CHIN and the patient record. The patient's record in the CHIN is comparable to a backup file for the patient's identification card.

A prescription ordered electronically will have followed the payer's formulary and preferred therapy guidelines. The prescriber will choose the drug from an electronic menu of product choices approved by the payer. The drugs will be in the inventory of network providers as assured by the manufacturer. As stated, drugs will be in unit of use packaging. Some will be starter packs to test results and tolerance; others will be maintenance packs. The packages will contain standardized drug information for the patient, thus satisfying one of the requirements now being sought by the FDA. Along with this drug information will be a compliance device for use by the patient. The pharmacist will instruct the patient on how to use the device. Some categories of drugs will have patient response cards or other means of recording scheduled health indicators. For example, antihypertensive drugs may have spaces for a patient to record periodic blood pressure readings and diabetic drugs places for blood glucose or other lab values.

Because these packages are bar coded and the prescription selected electronically, the dispensing individual will scan the product being dispensed. The scanner will validate that the bar code information in the computer for the drug matches the bar code information on the package. The chances of a dispensing error will be minimized.

When a prescription is delivered to a patient, the patient will turn over his or her identification card to have the transaction fulfilled. The pharmacist will be completing the delivery via an interactive video system. The patient's card will be "swiped" into a box that logs the patient onto the system. The pharmacist will have an identification card provided by the appropriate agency that contains all of the data regarding his or her professional status. This card will be used to log on the pharmacist with the patient. The patient will go through a drug/disease education process utilizing the video. The pharmacist will choose the literacy level for the patient and the required steps for the educational process. For example, a patient being treated for epilepsy will have to demonstrate a basic understanding of the disease as well as the drug. There can be a pretest to assess patient knowledge, or reference to information within the patient's file will indicate previous educational levels. The drug, dosage, side effects, etc., will be covered in detail, and at the end of the presentation, the patient will use the touch screen to record his or her answers in a permanent data file. The pharmacist will use this opportunity to update the patient's profile with any necessary changes in health status or with the addition of OTC purchases. If the patient was required to complete the previously discussed health response card, the pharmacist could enter the values of those indicators. All of this information would become resident in the health data bank.

Prescription refills will be handled in much the same manner. Patients will meet with the pharmacist to update their health status, report any problems, discuss compliance issues, etc.

This scenario for filling prescriptions answers many of the pressures now being applied to the retail pharmacy. The pharmacist will be paid not for the product, but for the outcome through intervention activities and the quality of the education provided. Logging on to the computer provides a record of the time spent, links the pharmacist with the patient, and accumulates the data for the outcome. In the future, payers will be less concerned with which pharmacy has the highest generic substitution ratio (savings due to reduced product cost) and more concerned with which pharmacy does the best job in patient compliance and reduced return visits to the physician (savings due to improved outcomes).

The level of pharmacy reimbursement will be contingent on the pharmacist's ability to successfully manage patients. This success will depend on several factors. We can assume that the quality of the educational materials will be controlled by the payer. Therefore, each pharmacist in a particular network will be using the same video presentation. Successful patient management will be differentiated through individual strengths in dealing with people and through professional expertise. Interpersonal skills in communication, in caring, and in teaching will become increasingly important.

Another difference in reimbursement will be in the drugs assigned to the network pharmacy. We previously discussed the expense of future biotech drugs and how it would be economically advisable to limit their distribution. Beyond inventory cost, think of the loss if the drug were being used improperly or inappropriately. It seems feasible to suggest that pharmacies would have to be qualified to receive and dispense these drugs. A physician prescribing these drugs would be directed to a menu that listed pharmacies authorized to inventory and dispense them. Pharmacists at these locations would be required to certify their level of knowledge related to the drug and to the disease state for which it is used. Arguably, we have a model for this in the Clozaril® system.

Which gets us back to the pharmacist's identification card. This card will be encoded with professional qualifications. Much like the idea that not every pharmacy will carry every drug, every pharmacist may or may not be accepted to educate a patient on every drug. The opportunity to be qualified and stay qualified will be available, but in this rapidly changing environment, securing a degree and a license will not convey life-long privileges for all professional activities. Neither is this idea far-fetched. We already have specialty licensing for various practice segments of pharmacy. This will only add skill levels within those segments.

A prescription transaction will be considered fulfilled when the patient receives the education along with the medication. When the pharmacist concludes the session, all electronic records are updated and the manufacturer is notified for inventory replenishment.

Technicians will perform the actual prescription-filling duties. Safety is assured by all of the electronic coding and safety checks done by scanning, as well as the fact that the pharmacist demonstrated the product, explained how to use the compliance card, recorded lab values, etc. Efficiency in the dispensing process will be enhanced by unit of use packaging. Today's time-consuming activity of making little bottles of pills from big bottles of pills will virtually cease to exist.

Replenishment will come from a local depot chosen by the manufacturer. The most logical facility to assume that role for independent pharmacy is today's wholesaler. The wholesaler will be linked to the network and will be responsible for the inventory control in the network stores. They will know which pharmacies are eligible for which drugs, dating on drugs shipped, damaged returns, and transfer of inventory. The drug wholesale industry seems to be tailor-made for such a purpose. Wholesalers have already gone through a consolidation process and have successfully transformed themselves into information and distribution specialists. Their expertise in systems management may make them a choice for maintaining the network support in terms of computer capabilities. Chains operate today very much like wholesalers and may continue to provide their own network support and pharmacy replenishment.

Not all drugs used by patients within a network will be dispensed on prescriptions. As discussed, payers will continue to work toward keeping people out of the system by placing emphasis on primary care. It follows that there will be a role for a professional who can control and dispense a third class of drugs. Whether these will be paid for by the network will depend on the drugs within this class. If there were clearly an economic savings to the payer through circumventing a physician visit, the drug would be covered. Once again, the health professional involved would have been certified to perform this function.

## MARKETING TO THE NEEDS
## OF THE FUTURE RETAIL PHARMACY

Regardless of whether, or how fast, we may ever see the scenario develop as described, there are certain irrefutable needs that will face the retail pharmacist. The primary one is assistance in the pharmacist's expanding involvement in the patient care process. All of the evidence suggests that there is a role for a health professional to fulfill the duties as described above for a retail pharmacy. But none of the evidence indicates a guarantee that the health professional will be a pharmacist. The key to such a guarantee is ensuring that the pharmacists engaged in retail practice can deliver the patient care required within an economically justifiable cost to the payer.

A simplified formula for retail pharmacy's economic cost to a payer would be the sum total of its location (convenience to the payer's subscribers), its systems capabilities (computer technology sufficient to participate), price for dispensing (cost of product plus agreed upon fee), and the expertise of the practitioners (drug product selection, DUR interventions, controlling outcomes). Successful marketing to the retail pharmacy segment, then, would be to concentrate efforts on each of these elements.

Helping retail pharmacy relative to location would include site selection for new locations and demographic analysis in older locations. Chain pharmacies possess their own formulas for deciding on a site. Independents are offered assistance through wholesalers. For both, it would seem that the strategy would be one of positioning to be able to participate in network coverage. Independents may look to find a site in a small community–one too small to support a chain–where a network may need a pharmacy. Aligning themselves with or nearby a medical facility should also improve independents' chances of being included within a network.

Demographic analysis for older locations would be used to target niche markets. Niche marketing relies on the maxim that successful providers of any product reside on either side of a volume scale: there is good profit in being a niche provider on the low-volume, high-margin end of the scale or good profit in being on the high-volume, low-margin end. The least profitable providers are those that reside toward the middle of the scale, making neither enough margin nor enough volume to survive very long. Marketers might consider using demographic analysis to evaluate the opportunity of converting certain retail locations to experts in a particular field of patient care. This would be a continuation but calculated enlargement of the way retailers currently jump into "hot new areas" such as home infusion and compounding. The advantage of the analysis and focus on specialization may have a twofold benefit. Pharmacists would expand their patient base while they are moving toward an expertise that would help satisfy the certification requirements of the future.

While discussing locations, it is interesting to speculate on what might happen to mail service pharmacies. If product cost is negotiated between a payer and a manufacturer, then mail service would no longer have a low cost advantage. The use of unit of use packaging and the need to guarantee education of the patient would seem to add to the savings limitations of mail service. In fact, shipping costs from mail service would add to the delivery expense.

Systems capabilities for retail pharmacies are a particularly onerous problem. Pharmacies make a significant investment when they choose a system, both in capital and in the requirement of human activities. Once a system is in place, customers become accustomed to what it will and will not deliver, and the users establish a comfort zone within its functionality. Changing systems becomes traumatic if not prohibitive. The ideal system will be one that provides flexibility, allows for expansion, recognizes patient care needs, and would be able to accommodate any payer network or CHIN requirements. A short list for marketers would include:

- Scanning capability used to identify patient, prescription, and product
- Data collection on patient care activities. Pharmacies should be able to receive a periodic report that indicates such data as how many times a prescription was not filled or was changed because of therapeutic problems.
- Data collection on physician activities. Pharmacies should be able to identify prescribers who are consistently outside of payer program guidelines for intervention.
- Receiving refill requests via a voice response unit

- Automatic printing of drug information for patients
- The ability to preset activity cues such as a refill reminder system
- Automatic calculation of compliance percentage for refills
- Access to drug product information and interactions
- Disease state management parameters.

This approach to systems needs is strictly health care focused. Pharmacy systems will have to be patient care systems and not carry the extra baggage of accounting, inventory control, and business activities. The pharmacy system will communicate necessary information to a business system.

Marketing to pricing concerns includes looking at both product cost and the cost for dispensing. Enough has been said previously about product cost and the current dilemma of multitiered pricing and rebates. If we do move to direct pricing for product, dispensing costs will be related to time spent with patients on health education and compliance issues. Marketing efforts that enhance these processes would be in order. An example might be for manufacturers to ensure that physician, pharmacist, and patient are using the same information and education source. When a physician is detailed on a prescription product, he or she should be shown the type of counseling information that the patient will receive at a pharmacy. Surely, every pharmacist has received a phone call from an irate prescriber who wants to know why the patient was given a specific warning of which the prescriber was unaware. Another example would be the design of material that would involve the patient in personal disease management. Marketing programs of this nature should emphasize helping the pharmacist to expand his or her role in patient involvement. Programs that attempt to enroll patients in a disease state support group must work with the pharmacist, not usurp the role.

The final item in our list of pharmacist's needs is to ensure the pharmacist's expertise within the rapidly changing boundaries of the profession. All marketing students are familiar with the life cycle of a product. It is born, grows within the marketplace to maturity, then declines. For long-term survival, it needs to be given new life–reinvented, if you will–during the maturity phase. If not, new and better products will replace it, ensuring its demise.

We can pose the analogy that pharmacy is a product that serves health care. It is in the process of reinventing itself. It is looking at its core competencies and depending on them for growth. It appears that the primary competency being universally singled out is the knowledge of drug product in managing patient care. We need to grow this ability, and growth in any endeavor requires continuous improvement.

I don't intend to enter into the debate over whether we should have mandatory Pharm.D. degrees. The type of graduate that is produced is not the issue. The issue is how we devise a controlled, continuous method to grow the abilities of those pharmacists already in practice. This is a step beyond mandated continuing education programs for relicensing. It implies the opportunity for a practicing pharmacist to maintain parity with recent graduates. Without such a system, even today's Pharm.D. graduates will face obsolescence in tomorrow's practice setting.

The need for this type of structured program through agreed upon educational resources and a single approving authority is already being felt in the third-party area. At the time of this writing, there are already several proposals for "credentialing" pharmacists, none of which are being validated by a central authority. The obvious problem here is that pharmacy will be overwhelmed by any number of payers who demand that dispensing pharmacists within a payer's network receive that payer's "credentialing."

For example, of the several programs mentioned, one charges from $6,000 to $10,000 for what appears to be an extensive package. It includes a computer system, remodeling, and training. This program will work with a college of pharmacy to measure the value of the program and develop a payment system that can be offered to payers. Yet another intends only to use a two-day live CE program, after which participants are deemed "credentialed." There is apparently no assessment before or after the program or any future measurement of the effectiveness of the seminar. There is a $200 fee per pharmacist for the "credentialing," and there may or may not be future programs required to maintain status. There is the promised possibility of higher reimbursement for "credentialed" providers (the implication that failure to enroll in the program will result in reduced reimbursements). It would seem that this particular program is merely an activity to generate more revenue for the plan sponsors.

Many manufacturers perform a valuable service in their current educational efforts and deserve our thanks for their assistance. They should be encouraged to continue their support. Marketers might enhance this support by joining these efforts to new product introduction. For example, rather than introduce a product through detailing, introduce it along with an approved continuing education program. Because these programs require fair balance in subject matter, pharmacists would have an opportunity to update their knowledge of disease state management each time a product is introduced.

I began this article with a quotation from Eric Hoffer. His was an interesting life. Born at the turn of the century, he had vision problems and was unable to read until his teenage years. He quickly caught up on his literacy and read everything–in English and German–he could get his hands on. He was a migrant worker, an Okie and an Arkie. He eventually settled on the Pacific coast, where he chose to work as a longshoreman so he could continue his passion for reading and observing human nature. He published books as collections of aphorisms, one of which is the quotation I used. Written about 40 years ago, it sounds as if it was intended to characterize the changes in today's health care market. While we cannot be certain about our future, we can be certain that we are being pushed into it rapidly. We can attempt to measure the direction we are being driven by examining the forces propelling us. What I have written is my own guess as to that future. Hopefully, it has provided some basis for your own thoughts.

# Independent Pharmacy:
# Rising to Meet the Challenge of the Future

Alicia S. Bouldin
John P. Bentley
D. C. Huffman
Dewey D. Garner

The independent community pharmacy has been an active presence on the corners of America's city streets for over a century. During that time, the independent's turf has expanded from main streets to include medical clinics and plazas, shopping centers, and urban neighborhoods. Throughout the course of this career, independents have seen many changes: from the rise to the demise of the soda fountain, from the restriction of counseling to the requirement of it, and from no required college curriculum to the six years of courses now being required in many states (up to two of those years in clinical training). Although the surrounding environment has changed, the independent pharmacist has always survived and has made his or her services available to the public.

Alicia S. Bouldin, B.S., is Research Assistant and AFPE Fellow; John P. Bentley, M.B.A., is Research Assistant and AFPE Fellow; and Dewey D. Garner, Ph.D., is Professor and Chair, all in the Department of Pharmacy Administration, School of Pharmacy, University of Mississippi, University, MS 38677. D. C. Huffman, Ph.D., is Executive Director of the NARD Management Institute and Senior Vice President for Pharmacy Practice and Management Services at NARD.

[Haworth co-indexing entry note]: "Independent Pharmacy: Rising to Meet the Challenge of the Future." Bouldin, Alicia S. et al. Co-published simultaneously in *Journal of Pharmaceutical Marketing & Management* (Pharmaceutical Products Press, an imprint of The Haworth Press, Inc.) Vol. 10, No. 2/3, 1996, pp. 149-166; and: *Pharmaceutical Marketing in the 21st Century* (ed: Mickey C. Smith) Pharmaceutical Products Press, an imprint of The Haworth Press, Inc., 1996, pp. 149-166. Single or multiple copies of this article are available from The Haworth Document Delivery Service [1-800-342-9678, 9:00 a.m. - 5:00 p.m. (EST)].

The *Lilly Digest* has revealed increases in gross sales for independent pharmacies for 44 consecutive years (1). Although the last 10 years have shown a trend in decreasing gross margins, independent pharmacists have met that challenge. They have done this in part by operating more efficiently, as revealed by the trend in decreasing total expenses for those same 10 years, maintaining their before-tax net profit at around 3% of sales (with the exception of 1992, when profit was only 1.9%). The 1994 edition of the *NARD-Lilly Digest* indicated that prescription sales had increased 16.3% over the previous year, suggesting that independents are maintaining their share of the prescription pie, even in the face of competition and third-party restrictions (1).

Community pharmacy is thriving, and the independent pharmacist who is willing to adapt to the changes now occurring in our health care system will also thrive. The role of the pharmacist is changing as the paradigm of practice shifts from functions centered primarily on dispensing to functions whose center is more patient-focused (2). Some of the important contributions pharmacists are capable of making to the quality of patient care have been recognized. Part of this recognized shift in focus has been driven by legislation such as OBRA 90, which mandated counseling and drug use review for Medicaid beneficiaries. The shift of focus to the patient has also been motivated by the patients themselves. Today's consumer is often better educated regarding medications than the consumer of even ten years ago. This is thanks to the ready availability of medical information and to the education and promotion provided by the pharmaceutical manufacturers, who seized the opportunity to "speak" to this empowered consumer through promotion aimed directly at the consumer. With tomorrow's promise of an information explosion and abundant travel on the information superhighway, the consumer of the future will require perhaps not more, but different, types of attention from pharmacists as primary health care professionals.

The intricacy of drug regimens for today's patient requires the transference of pharmacy practice characteristics instituted in the hospital to the community setting, from simpler functions such as monitoring drug therapy to more detailed functions such as initiating and altering therapy. The term pharmaceutical care has been receiving considerable attention, both in the language of the health professions and now among lay persons as well. Pharmacists are aware that embracing the idea of pharmaceutical care may require modification of the way many view their roles and expansion of those roles to include as commonplace some skills that pharmacists have had little opportunity to demonstrate in the past. This extended concept of care is not likely to go away as we move into the next century, but will almost certainly grow in the future.

Computerization has in one sense liberated community pharmacists from some of the labors that once enslaved them. Because of the advanced record-keeping, billing, and on-line information search capabilities of computers, the pharmacist has more time to spend in patient-oriented services. Thus, technology has provided a potential strength to the independent pharmacist, if he or she learns to master the machine and to make good use of the liberty it provides, in patient care and perhaps in entrepreneurial pursuits.

The future of independent community pharmacy rests in the ability of its practitioners to capitalize on its strengths and to take full advantage of the opportunities that exist, emphasizing service over product.

## THE STRENGTH OF INDEPENDENT PHARMACY

Communities across the United States have long depended upon their local family pharmacist for medication, advice, and support. But nowhere is that dependence upon the pharmacist's services more prominent than in our nation's small towns and rural areas. In these areas, the independent pharmacist is not only a respected entrepreneur, but also the primary resident health care professional. For decades, the driving force behind the provision of pharmaceutical services in these pharmacies has been necessity. Here is an example.

In Sledge, Mississippi (population 350), independent pharmacist Luck Wing operated a community pharmacy for approximately 40 years, practicing pharmacy for the first of those decades with only an occasional visit by a physician to the town he served. In that isolation, Mr. Wing became an invaluable resource for the community. Not only did he meet the medication needs of the people in Sledge, but he also attempted to serve them anywhere he saw an unmet need. He provided a bridal registry for his community, making china patterns available. He carpeted his pharmacy with indoor-outdoor carpet and established a carpet franchise within his store. He made keys. He even provided veterinary injections for the pets of the town (3). This symbiosis aided his own financial standing and enabled him to remain in business, while providing the much-needed services he offered to his customers. The motivation to serve where opportunity and need exist has been a strength of the independent's practice from the beginning.

Another strength of independent pharmacy which the consumer has always realized is the personal attention given to the customer. Researchers have found that the elderly appreciate the "personal touch" and may seek that personal factor over convenience (4). The community pharmacy that capitalizes on this population's need for services (drug information, consultation, delivery) will find a competitive edge over the pharmacy that does not make these services satisfactorily available. Lip service will not suffice for a significant portion of the population. As the population is graying with the baby boomers and beyond, the development of this strength of independent pharmacy may be a necessary factor for growth in the future.

Community pharmacists have found strength in numbers through NARD, Representing Independent Retail Pharmacy. Since its beginnings in 1898 as the National Association of Retail Druggists, NARD has been the voice of the independent and has made the independent's goals, needs, and interests known to other associations, to legislators, and to the public (5). The American College of Apothecaries (ACA) educates, maintains the standards, and guards the interests of those pharmacists whose practices are limited to health-related products and services and who practice the specialized art of compounding.

Even with these strengths in hand, independent pharmacy must keep a keen weather eye on the changes occurring around it–in the marketplace, in the legislature, and in the patient's perspective. Without global vision, independents may find it difficult to adapt to the dynamic environment that surrounds them. No strength can compensate for an inability to change.

## THE CHANGING MARKETPLACE

The community pharmacy marketplace, once characterized by minimal competition among many small, owner-operated independent pharmacies, has changed dramatically during the past 20 years (6). With these changes, independent pharmacies have had to alter their business practices to survive and to compete. Changes in the community pharmacy marketplace and in the health care environment in general have presented independent pharmacies with a number of threats and challenges to their existence, while at the same time revealing a number of opportunities to increase their presence and profits.

### Challenges

While there are several challenges facing the health care industry in general (i.e., health care reform legislation), some of these are specific to the community pharmacy marketplace. One significant challenge to independent pharmacies is competition. A decade ago, the primary competitors for independent pharmacies were chain pharmacies, which rapidly gained market share in the 1960s and 1970s. The 1980s ushered in a number of new competitors: supermarkets and mass merchandisers began to open pharmacy departments; health maintenance organizations began to provide pharmaceutical services through in-house pharmacies; and mail-order pharmacies grew rapidly during this time period, primarily through contracts with large employers.

Even with all forms of competition included, independent pharmacies comprise the largest single component of the pharmacy market on the basis of number of stores (7, 8). Although a decrease in the number of independent pharmacies has occurred during recent years, independent pharmacies increased their purchases through wholesalers by 9% in 1993, an increase consistent with other competitors in the marketplace (7). The pharmacy failure rate is significantly less than that of small businesses in general (9). Independent pharmacies continue to derive the majority of their total sales from prescriptions. The 1994 *NARD-Lilly Digest* revealed that prescription income accounted for 79.4% of total sales in these pharmacies (1).

Another challenge encountered by independent pharmacies and the community pharmacy marketplace in general has been the rapid growth of third-party prescription plans. These programs paid for only 18.5% of the total number of prescriptions dispensed in community pharmacies in 1972 (10). Cost-containment efforts of the 1980s and 1990s dramatically increased this percentage so that by 1993, third parties (Medicaid and other third parties) accounted for about 50% of prescriptions dispensed in the retail setting (7). In fact, in the fourth quarter of 1993, third-party payment surpassed cash as the leading method of payment for retail prescriptions (7). The future status of the independent's relationship with third-party programs may be dubious. A study conducted by Carroll using differential analysis to forecast and examine the impact of the growth of third-party prescription programs on the profitability of independent pharmacies showed that many pharmacies may have increased short-term profits by participating in third-party programs but that the long-term effects of increased third-party coverage (given current trends and assumptions) will be detrimental to pharmacy profits (11).

Pharmaceutical benefit managers (PBMs) have also raised concerns for independents. These organizations contract with employers, insurers, PPOs, IPA managed care plans, network model managed care plans, and (increasingly) HMOs to handle the pharmacy benefits of their enrollees.

Medicaid agencies have also begun to contract with these specialized firms. Services provided by PBMs may include benefit design, claims administration, drug distribution (through pharmacy networks and/or mail services), MACs, formularies, and drug use management (12).

Plans managed by PBMs are covering an increasing number of prescriptions. In an effort to cut costs, these organizations (in addition to other providers of pharmaceutical benefits) offer pharmacies contracts with small dispensing fees. Some PBMs are also offering benefits to their enrollees through closed networks from which some pharmacies are excluded. Thus, independents are often placed in a difficult position: they are excluded from even participating in some plans, and the plans in which they do participate provide them with a decreasing level of reimbursement for their services. In addition to the reductions in reimbursement level by PBMs and other third-party payers, the four-year moratorium on reducing Medicaid pharmacy reimbursements expired in December of 1994, "thus freeing state legislators to target these reimbursements as a way to trim overall Medicaid costs" (13).

### Opportunities

While PBMs have considerably altered the environment, the growing influence of these organizations may actually have a positive impact on independent pharmacies (12). Some PBMs are developing programs to compensate pharmacists for complying with formulary management and therapeutic recommendation programs. Additionally, as will be discussed later, the reimbursement of pharmacists by PBMs (and other providers of pharmacy benefits) for the provision of cognitive services offers independent pharmacies a significant opportunity to achieve professional satisfaction while increasing revenue (14).

In addition to the potential of reimbursement to pharmacists for cognitive services, several other changes are occurring that present independent pharmacists with opportunities. Porter has outlined two "generic" strategies for outperforming other organizations in a particular industry: lower cost and differentiation (15). These two strategies can be applied to a broad target (cost leadership and differentiation) or a narrow target (cost focus and focused differentiation). By acting on opportunities presented, independent pharmacies have the potential to differentiate themselves from their competitors, thus gaining a competitive advantage. Several trends continue to shape the community pharmacy marketplace, providing opportunities for entrepreneurial pharmacists to seize. Some of these trends include: an aging population, biotechnology (high tech), individual service (high touch), a movement toward self-care, reduction of time being spent in the hospital setting, and changes in illness patterns toward chronic debilitating illness.

Individuals over the age of 65 comprise approximately 12% of the total U.S. population but account for 30% of total health expenditures (16). Additionally, this segment of the population consumes 30% of all prescription drugs and 40% of all OTC products (16). Over 85% of the ambulatory elderly and 95% of those living in nursing homes use medication on a regular basis (17). This older segment of the population is expected to continue to grow well into the next century. Noncompliance and adverse drug reactions are well documented in this population. These trends have had and should continue to have a significant impact on community pharmacy practice. One implication for these trends is the increased involvement of pharmacists in long-term care facilities. Independent pharmacists are very active in this market segment. According to the 1994 *NARD-Lilly Digest,* 35% of members provide services to long-term care facilities (1). Another implication for these trends is discussed above: the "personal touch" aspect of care. In his best-seller, *Megatrends,* John Naisbitt proposes that "whenever there is a new technology introduced into society, there must be a counterbalancing human response (i.e., high touch) or the technology is rejected" (18). As pharmaceuticals and medicine continue to become more high tech and as the population continues to age, there will be a need for a high-touch medical professional. Independent pharmacists are in the optimal position to fill that need.

Bezold predicts that the next two decades will see steady growth in the amount of self-care and dramatic improvement in the quality of that care for most individuals in Europe and the U.S. (19). He outlines several trends that are driving the self-care movement: a new attitude toward health, including increased self-responsibility for health; a growing aging population with a new attitude toward aging that stresses more healthy, "successful aging" and "compression of morbidity"; ever-expanding biomedical knowledge; the development of very effective expert systems for diagnosis and treatment and their use in self-care books and software used by consumers; electronic medical records; and cost and other pressures toward optimal cost-effective care which will lead physicians and health care providers to enhance the home self-care of their patients. The self-care movement will likely have a dramatic impact not only on independent pharmacy but also on the relationship between independent pharmacists and their patients. Consumers are demanding more information, and the independent pharmacist is in a position to provide that information. Additionally, OTC product counseling has become more important in the age of consumerism, and the Rx-to-OTC switch raises the issue of a third-class of pharmacy-only drug products.

Several challenges and opportunities await independent pharmacy due to the changing marketplace. To sum up these changes and the place of independent pharmacy in the future of the marketplace, Charles M. West, Executive Vice President of NARD, offers this statement, quoted in an article appearing in the January 1995 issue of *American Druggist*: "There will always be independent pharmacies. There may not be quite as many, but there will be a substantial number. They'll probably be bigger and more efficient, but there will always be independent pharmacies" (20).

## THE INDEPENDENT'S RESPONSE
## TO THE CHANGING MARKETPLACE

As the marketplace whittles away at the dispensing fee and forces down profit margins industrywide, community pharmacists are attempting to demonstrate the value of their services. One reason for the past reluctance of third-party payers to reimburse pharmacists for such services has been the lack of an operational definition of value-added services (21). Most authors have failed to distinguish between the professional services expected in dispensing a prescription and other services that are important aspects of providing pharmaceutical care (14).

Christensen and colleagues describe pharmaceutical care as incorporating three components (21). These three components correspond to three categories of cognitive services: dispensing services, dispensing-related services, and non-dispensing-related value-added services. Dispensing services include accurately filling a prescription order, clarifying incomplete or illegible prescriptions, not dispensing orders that a reasonable and prudent pharmacist would recognize as containing obvious errors, and communicating drug use instructions to patients as required by applicable regulations. These are considered basic services and are usually covered within the dispensing fee.

Dispensing-related services include monitoring patient use of drugs; detecting less than optimal therapy; and consulting with the prescriber, the patient, or other health providers. Two dispensing-related value-added services have recently received a considerable amount of attention from researchers, industry representatives, and pharmacists: therapeutic recommendations and compliance programs. Many independents have recognized the opportunities present and have involved themselves with these types of activities.

As described by Banahan and colleagues, retail pharmacists appear to be taking a more active role in the drug selection process by intervening after prescriptions are written (22). While the literature is inconsistent with respect to definitions, this activity is generally referred to as therapeutic recommendation, defined as "a suggestion to a patient, the prescribing physician, or both to change a prescription to a therapeutically equivalent but generically inequivalent drug" (14). When a physician accepts the recommendation, the pharmacist records the new prescription and dispenses the alternative product. These recommendations may occur because of clinical and/or economic reasons.

This activity has been well documented in recent years. One study found that 79% of independent pharmacists indicated that they make therapeutic recommendations to physicians that prescriptions be changed to an alternative, equivalent drug product because of the high cost of the medication prescribed (23). This percentage, representing the independent's involvement, was significantly higher than the percentage of chain pharmacists making such recommendations (69%) (23). In a more recent study, retail pharmacists reported that they make 6.1 therapeutic recommendations each week and physicians reportedly accept 81.4% of recommendations made (22). Economic reasons, such as patient price concerns and the availability of more economical products, are the main issues currently stimulating therapeutic recommendations (22). While economic concerns will always be with us, clinical issues will continue to grow in importance as pharmacists continue to perform drug utilization review activities.

The pharmaceutical industry is in a unique position concerning therapeutic recommendations and interventions. Pharmacists generally feel that they should be compensated for these activities, "but are not completely comfortable with the prospect of being rewarded for these interventions by pharmaceutical companies" (22). This is especially true for programs that reimburse pharmacists for successfully switching patients to a sponsored product. An alternative for pharmaceutical companies desiring involvement with this dispensing-related aspect of pharmacy practice could include working through managed care organizations or PBMs to minimize the potential conflict of interest (22).

Another dispensing-related service that pharmacists can provide for their patients is compliance monitoring/intervention. Numerous studies have demonstrated that compliance with medications is poor. Research has suggested that 30%-75% of patients do not adequately comply with the treatment suggested by the physician. This figure is reported by some to approach 90% (24). Noncompliance has a potentially negative impact not only on patients but also on pharmacies, manufacturers, and society. Because of their access to records and their role in patient counseling, pharmacists are in an ideal position to have a positive effect on patient compliance.

In a small study conducted by *American Druggist,* 32.8% of independent pharmacies reported that they maintained an ongoing compliance program (25). Additionally, manufacturers have recently initiated a number of programs designed to improve patient compliance. For the most part, manufacturers have attempted to involve pharmacists in these programs. Although the benefit to the patient may exist, manufacturers need to be aware of the potential negative consequences of these programs. In a study recently completed, researchers found that "pharmacists believed that patient programs are substantially more valuable for the companies that develop them than they are for patients, who are the targets, and pharmacists, the program facilitators" (26).

The final category of cognitive services defined by Christensen and colleagues is non-dispensing-related services. These include such services as training patients to use blood glucose monitoring devices and providing academic detailing. Many of the services that independent pharmacists have long been providing can be classified as non-dispensing-related services. Blood pressure screening, cholesterol screening, and other health screening and promotional activities are fairly commonplace in community pharmacies. Diabetes care centers and nutritional services are being provided by an increasing number of pharmacists. Many of these non-dispensing-related services may be viewed as entrepreneurial opportunities that independent pharmacies must capitalize upon to remain viable in the highly competitive community pharmacy marketplace. Thus, a recent response of the independent has been to seek reimbursement for the non-dispensing and value-added services they provide.

## PAYMENT FOR COGNITIVE SERVICES

The extent of involvement in these cognitive services has often depended on the pharmacist's comfort with his or her knowledge of the subject in question, the allowable time away from dispensing in a busy workday, and other such factors. The importance often placed on volume over care may make finding time to provide these services difficult for many pharmacists (27). However, with the changes in the marketplace described here (such as limits set on dispensing profit margins by third-party payers and government regulations) contributing to dwindling margins in the independent's business, pharmacists may need to rely more on cognitive services (for example, consultation with patients regarding medication and disease state, maintaining a patient medication profile and screening drug utilization, providing nutritional services and clinical services) for their independent pharmacies to remain viable and active businesses.

Cost savings is the major impetus behind managed care organizations, and in the case of pharmacy, that impetus has led to profit restrictions and a push for greater speed in dispensing (enter mail order). Receiving some notice, however, are the cost savings possible through the application of appropriate pharmacy services. Community pharmacists, recognizing the value of their own services to the health care system and seeing that value described by others, have been seeking reimbursement for those services. Although reimbursing the pharmacist for these services may cost the managed care organization, the value of the services may far outweigh their cost. And reimbursement to the pharmacist for these services encourages their continuation.

The three main reasons third-party administrators give for being reluctant to reimburse pharmacists for cognitive services are: it is too costly to reimburse, those services are the pharmacist's professional responsibility, and plan enrollees were satisfied already (28). Some administrators stated that they would pay for pharmacy services that improved patient satisfaction or decreased total costs. Pharmacists, therefore, must be able to demonstrate how eliminating symptoms affects the patient's satisfaction and how reduction of utilization and costs may result from cognitive services (28).

Pharmacy services can play a large role in controlling health care costs, especially with the increasing use of prescription medications and the increasing potential for Rx-to-OTC switches. The value of these services should not be overlooked. In the United States alone, noncompliance with therapeutic regimens causes an estimated 125,000 deaths every year and costs 20 million workdays and $1.5 billion in earnings per year (29). Noncompliance with antihypertensive medications is a serious problem which may cost $10,500 per year (double the cost for a compliant patient) and can result in required hospitalization (30). In fact, drug noncompliance accounts for 10% of hospital admissions and $8.5 billion in excess hospitalization annually (29). Studies show that between 8% and 13% of all hospitalizations result from inappropriate drug use. This includes incidences of overuse; underuse; and drug interactions, due in part to complex drug regimens; and the use of multiple prescribers and pharmacies (29). Much of this inappropriate drug use could be reduced by more widespread utilization of available pharmacy services. The cost of a single day in the hospital averages about $600, whereas the average prescription cost is slightly over $26 (1, 31). These figures may only increase in the coming years. Cognitive services provided by the community pharmacist, such as patient education and compliance screening of medication profiles, could help to curb these unnecessary costs of inappropriate drug use and continue to prove extremely relevant in this arena.

How can pharmacists' interventions reduce that potential cost from inappropriate drug use? In a study conducted by Dobie and colleagues, 47% of the instances in which pharmacists intervened regarding a problematic prescription held potential for harm to the patient from the prescribing errors committed. Most often, the medical care required to treat that harm was predicted by expert evaluators to be urgent care in the form of an unscheduled physician contact. However, that level of care was closely followed by "emergency medical attention with hospitalization likely" (31). Those potential additional costs merit the attention of plan administrators. If future studies show results consistent with these, there will be no room for doubt regarding the value added by the services a pharmacist can provide.

Although these value-added services cost the pharmacist time and therefore cost the pharmacist or payer money, the end value (better quality in patient care) is significantly greater than the up-front cost of the service. A 1988 study revealed that a pharmacist's intervention in a prescribing error cost about $1.75 per intervention at that time (based on a pharmacist salary of $15 per hour). But the mean value of each intervention (in costs avoided) was estimated at $7.15, which represented a value-to-cost ratio of 4 to 1 (32). Those figures merit the attention of administrators interested in cost savings.

At present, third-party billing for cognitive services requires documentation of need for the service, as well as documentation that the service was delivered. It is suggested that claims for reimbursement include a cover letter, a certificate of medical necessity (describing the type of consultation deemed necessary by the physician), the pharmacotherapeutic consultation report, and an invoice for the services (28, 33). These types of communication now require time, effort, and paperwork. However, as technology progresses to allow further networking among all players on the health care team–physician, pharmacist, payer, and patient–this process may become simpler and therefore more acceptable.

A consultation report filled out after the service has been provided serves as evidence of the consultation and allows the third party to have a record of the service for which it is paying. Currently, creative pharmacists are using a variety of forms to document the consultation (including the NARD Pharmacist Care Claim Form) in order to file for reimbursement.

Michael T. Rupp, associate professor at Purdue University's School of Pharmacy and Pharmacal Sciences, states that uniformity in the form of a nationally recognized standard for documentation and transmission of cognitive services is needed for routine reimbursement (34). This is perhaps one of the greatest barriers now existing to obtaining reimbursement. Pharmacist orders for more than 250,000 NARD Pharmacist Care Claim Forms indicate a desire to use these forms to provide standardized documentation of the services pharmacists provide in hope that the value realized from these pharmacy services may lead to reimbursement. Presenting third parties with a system similar to that which they are already using successfully–such as a standard set of billing categories as widely recognized as the ICD-9 and CPT codes used by physicians–would almost certainly enhance the process of reimbursement to pharmacists for their services, and the National Council for Prescription Drug Programs is currently developing these codes (35).

The technology of the future may make on-line invoicing widespread, similar to electronic submission of prescription claims for adjudication. Already an invoice designed by Bill Felkey and others for documentation of both the intervention and the estimated value of the service has been computerized for on-line use for independent pharmacists in the CogniCare system of CarePoint in South Carolina. Invoices may be submitted on the same equipment that carries claims, simplifying the reimbursement process and making it more feasible (35). The future holds much promise for such electronic transfer and submission.

Some cognitive services provide much in the way of preventive care: screening, counseling, and educating patients regarding their medications. However, pharmacy services have enormous potential in the area of prevention, and this potential is largely, as yet, untapped. One source has proposed that, in the future, pharmacists will be reimbursed for a wellness evaluation. Such an evaluation would last 20 to 30 minutes and might include immunization profiles, outcome evaluation, self-care counseling (OTCs), nutritional and general health counseling, and health risk appraisal, to name a few possibilities (36). Preventive care may play a much larger role after any reform of the health care system, as adequate prevention could be expected to save countless future health care dollars.

With the growing focus on quality of patient care, these services will be occupying more and more of the pharmacist's time. Establishing the idea of payment for these services now will have a significant impact on the way payment is viewed in the future. Therefore, how independent pharmacists deal with the issue of documenting the value of and seeking reimbursement for their cognitive services today may greatly influence the independent's business tomorrow.

While it is true that establishment of an acceptable system for reimbursing pharmacists for their nondispensing services will facilitate and encourage the continuation of those services, it must also be stated that reimbursement alone may not be the answer to the independent's challenge of maintaining a viable business. The pharmacist with an entrepreneurial spirit may find additional opportunities as the face of health care changes.

## *ENTREPRENEURIAL OPPORTUNITIES*

In the past, independent pharmacies have relied primarily on differentiation strategies to gain a competitive advantage. One of those strategies has been differentiation through customer service, including delivery services and store charge systems. Additionally, independents have employed the strategy of providing other, non-dispensing-related specialty services, including diabetes education, service to long-term care facilities, home health care equipment and home infusion supplies and services, specialized compounding services, nutrition services and counseling, homeopathic medicines (stocking them) and consultation on their use, hospice service and involvement in pain management, ostomy and wound care, respiratory therapy consulting, patient fittings for orthotic and prosthetic supplies, health screening and promotion, and immunizations.

To recognize the potential for these services, independent pharmacies must constantly scan their environments for opportunities. A good example of how environmental scanning may lead to the development of a new service by an independent pharmacy is the case of home infusion therapy. Due to cost-containment pressures and prospective payment systems, the average length of stay at a short-term acute care hospital declined significantly in the 1980s (Figure 1). The average length of stay at a short-term acute care community hospital declined to 7.1 days in 1992 from 7.6 days in 1980. This trend, coupled with a general societal trend toward self-care, led to an expansion of the home health care market. Additionally, it became increasingly recognized that some therapies such as chemotherapy and long-term IV antibiotic therapy could be performed in the home, and technological advancements are making this therapy more feasible. This led to the growth of the home IV market, which is expected to continue its rapid growth throughout the decade (Figure 2).

Independent pharmacies and pharmacists are providing a wide range of services that are "redefining their role on the health care team" (37). By

FIGURE 1. Average Length of Stay: Acute Care Hospital. .

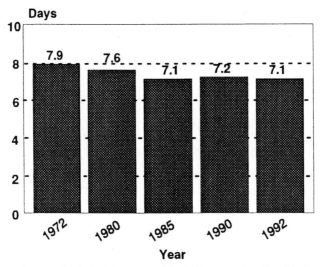

Source: Statistical Abstract of the U.S.: 1994 (114th edition)

attempting to differentiate themselves, independents are becoming more actively involved in managing patient drug therapy and outcomes, in addition to other aspects of their care.

## THE INDEPENDENT PHARMACY OF THE FUTURE

The changing role of the community pharmacist, the changing needs of the patient, and the changes looming on the horizon suggest that the practice of pharmacy will look different in the years to come. As the functions performed within tomorrow's independent pharmacy will almost certainly be different from those performed there today, the layout of the pharmacy will differ widely from the traditional design to which we are accustomed. Progress in automation and an emphasis on service will be reflected in a design that would allow more interaction between the pharmacist and the patient. The vastness and ready availability of information in multiple media will benefit both the pharmacist and the patient and will enhance the quality of each patient's care. No matter how far one might take the predicted picture of independent pharmacy in the 21st century, the most important ingredient in this independent pharmacy of the future is

FIGURE 2. Home IV Market: Projected Growth (1993-2000).

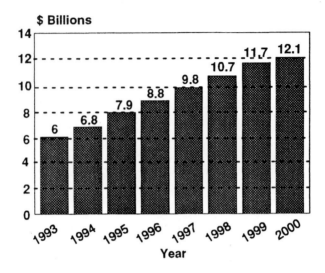

Source: The National Home Infusion Association

still the pharmacist, the person. What that independent pharmacist becomes depends upon the resiliency, the inventiveness, and the entrepreneurial spirit of the pharmacist as he or she enters this new era.

## REFERENCES

1. NARD. 1994 NARD-Lilly Digest.

2. Trinca CE. The pharmacist's progress towards implementing pharmaceutical care. Unpublished.

3. Smith MC. The view from Sledge. PM Pharm Manage J 1967;(Jul):13.

4. Anon. Serving the growing senior market. NARD J 1990;112(8):47-50.

5. Sonnedecker G, ed. Kremers and Urdang's history of pharmacy. 4th ed. Philadelphia: JB Lippincott, 1976.

6. Carroll NV, Jowdy AW. Demographic and prescription patronage motive differences among segments in the community pharmacy market. J Pharm Market Manage 1987;1(4):19-33.

7. Anon. Annual report: facts and figures. Drug Store News Pharm 1994;4(4):38.

8. NABP. 1994 NABP Survey of Pharmacy Law.

9. McKay AB. Entrepreneurship. NARD Management Institute course.

10. Anon. Third parties pay for 1 out of every 4 Rxs. Am Druggist 1975;172(2):56+.

11. Carroll NV. Forecasting the impact of participation in third-party prescription programs on pharmacy profits. J Res Pharm Econ 1991;3(3):3-23.

12. American Pharmaceutical Association. Opportunities for the community pharmacist in managed care. Washington, DC: American Pharmaceutical Association, 1994.

13. Biro S. Reimbursement to pharmacists has not increased Medicaid costs in past 10 years. Pharm Today 1995;1(4):22-3.

14. Banahan BF III, Basara LR. Therapeutic recommendations: the future of clinical community pharmacy practice. Am Druggist 1994;211(1):75-82.

15. Porter ME. The competitive advantage of nations. New York: The Free Press, 1990.

16. Gooen LG. Consultant pharmacy: an evolving practice. Pharm Times 1990;56(11):47-53.

17. Lipton HL. The graying of America: implications for the pharmacist. Am J Hosp Pharm 1982;39:131-5.

18. Naisbitt J. Megatrends: ten new directions transforming our lives. New York: Warner Books, 1984.

19. Bezold C. Future trends in self-medication and self-care. J Soc Admin Pharm 1990;7:205-15.

20. Holt C. Focusing on pharmacy's future: what things will look like in the year 2000. Am Druggist 1995;211(3):20-3.

21. Christensen DB, Fassett WE, Andrews GA. A practical billing and payment plan for cognitive services. Am Pharm 1993;NS33(3):34-40.

22. Banahan BF III, McCaffrey DJ III, Kolassa EM. Community pharmacists' attitudes toward and involvement in therapeutic recommendations and cognitive service reimbursement programs. University, MS: University of Mississippi, 1995.

23. Banahan BF III, McCaffrey DJ III. Pharmacists' growing influence on MDs' product selection. Pharm Times 1993;59(8):28-40.

24. Debrovner D. Did you take your pill today? Am Druggist 1992;206(6):60-6.

25. Anon. Flash point: pill patrol. Am Druggist 1992;206(6):60-6.

26. Basara LR, Smith MC. Community pharmacists' attitudes toward company sponsored patient programs. Unpublished.

27. Ukens C. Whatever happened to pharmaceutical care? Drug Top 1994;138 (5):38-52.

28. Summers K. Getting reimbursed for nondispensing services. Drug Top 1993;137 (17):74-86.

29. NARD news release: the costs and consequences of drug noncompliance.

30. Anon. Controlling health care costs through comprehensive pharmacy care. Alexandria, VA: NARD, 1992.

31. Dobie RL, Rascati KL. Documenting the value of pharmacist interventions. Am Pharm 1994;NS34(5):50-4.

32. Rupp MT. Evaluation of prescribing errors and pharmacist interventions in community practice: an estimate of "value added." Am Pharm 1988;NS28(12):22-6.

33. Meade V. Getting paid for cognitive services. Am Pharm 1994;NS34(6):32-6.

34. Cardinale V. Cognitive-pay movement gains momentum, APhA told. Drug Top 1994;138(8):79-80.

35. Felkey B, Schondelmeyer S, Berger B. Invoicing pharmacist interventions. Am Pharm 1994;NS34(6):37-8.

36. Rosendahl I. Preventive care: a promise of opportunity. Drug Top 1994;138 (1):42-52.

37. Anon. Independent pharmacy ownership: forging pharmacy's future. NARD J 1992;114(4):18-28.

# New Rules for Marketing Pharmaceuticals to Hospitals

Joseph A. Oddis
William A. Zellmer

## INTRODUCTION

The hospital industry and pharmacy practice in hospitals are undergoing profound changes. At the macro level, the hospital field is being realigned in three ways: in the relationships among hospitals, in the relationships between hospitals and other components of health care delivery, and in the relationships between hospitals and the purchasers of their services. At the micro level, the day-to-day activities of institutions are being reengineered to make them more responsive to patient needs. In addition to these changes, pharmacy practice is transforming itself through its shift to pharmaceutical care.

To prepare for successful marketing to hospitals in the future, pharmaceutical companies must understand these shifts and adjust their strategies to accommodate them. In this article, we elaborate on the three changes mentioned above and discuss their implications for drug companies.

## REALIGNMENT IN THE HOSPITAL INDUSTRY

Two trends are at work in the realignment of hospitals. The first trend, the creation of multihospital systems, has been at work for several years

Joseph A. Oddis, Sc.D., is Executive Vice President of the American Society of Health-System Pharmacists, 7272 Wisconsin Avenue, Bethesda, MD 20814. William A. Zellmer, M.P.H., is Vice President for Professional and Government Affairs at ASHP.

[Haworth co-indexing entry note]: "New Rules for Marketing Pharmaceuticals to Hospitals." Oddis, Joseph A., and William A. Zellmer. Co-published simultaneously in *Journal of Pharmaceutical Marketing & Management* (Pharmaceutical Products Press, an imprint of The Haworth Press, Inc.) Vol. 10, No. 2/3, 1996, pp. 167-176; and: *Pharmaceutical Marketing in the 21st Century* (ed: Mickey C. Smith) Pharmaceutical Products Press, an imprint of The Haworth Press, Inc., 1996, pp. 167-176. Single or multiple copies of this article are available from The Haworth Document Delivery Service [1-800-342-9678, 9:00 a.m. - 5:00 p.m. (EST)].

and has recently accelerated through the construction of large chains of investor-owned (for-profit) hospitals. The second trend, the creation of integrated health care systems or networks, is a more recent phenomenon, spawned in part by the failure of federal health care reform.

Following World War II, the federal government adopted a policy of expanding the number of hospitals, with the goal of making acute-care services more accessible to all citizens. The postwar growth in employer-funded hospital insurance, the passage of Medicare, and federal support of specialty medical training greatly fueled overall expansion of the hospital field. Money was readily available for facility construction and for the expensive diagnostic and treatment technology used in those facilities. It gradually became clear that this push for hospital expansion went too far, driving up costs at an alarming rate.

As national policy toward hospital care moved from the accelerator to the brake, financial resources for acute care became scarcer. One response of hospitals was to merge in an attempt to achieve various efficiencies, such as in management, access to capital, application of high technology, and purchase of supplies. ASHP's 1994 survey of hospital pharmacies indicated that 43% of institutions were members of multihospital systems (1).

A deeper realignment of hospitals is of more recent origin, namely, the creation of integrated health care systems or networks. This development is the private sector response to national health care reform. Employers, who fund a large proportion of health care, continue to seek more effective mechanisms to control the cost of health care for their workers. Health care providers concluded that they needed to find more effective ways of organizing their services so that they could be more competitive in bidding on employer contracts. It appears as though the needs of both purchasers and providers have converged to foster the creation of integrated health care systems.

Integrated systems bring together providers (typically, at the start, hospitals and physician group practices) in the creation of new organizations that contract with employers and insurance companies to provide care on a per capita fee basis. Often, an insurance company or an HMO is a partner in the organization. Because the organization contracts to provide the agreed-upon level of care for a fixed price per enrollee, it has a powerful, self-imposed incentive to plan and manage its resources wisely. This incentive is expected to be far more effective in rationalizing resource consumption than externally imposed utilization review. The theory that integrated systems will produce effective cost control in health care depends, of course, on the existence of competing systems within particular health care markets.

The leader in the creation of an integrated health care system is generally a hospital, a large group medical practice, a hospital-physician organization, or an insurance company (2). Mature integrated systems have incorporated home care and long-term care in addition to acute care and ambulatory care. A major challenge for integrated systems is the coordination of care across practice sites, which will require a heavy investment in information systems.

In the 1994 ASHP hospital pharmacy survey, 61% of hospitals had "made deliberate moves toward becoming part of an integrated health care system" (1). For purposes of the survey, integrated systems were defined as organizational arrangements "in which patients can receive all levels and types of health care services from affiliated provider organizations with coordinated case management and interprovider information flow."

We expect that pharmacy practice in all components of integrated health care systems will eventually have many characteristics similar to those of hospital pharmacy today. For example, pharmacists will work in close cooperation with other members of the health care team, providing the benefit of their knowledge of drug therapy, both in the care of individual patients and in the formulation of drug use policies.

The management opportunities for pharmacists in integrated health care systems are exciting, and many current hospital pharmacy department directors will find themselves in those roles. To be successful in this new environment, however, the pharmacy director will have to learn new ways of thinking. In particular, the traditional focus of the director on controlling the hospital's drug budget will have to be replaced with a broader pharmacoeconomic and outcomes perspective. The focus must be on determining which products will achieve the best overall results for the patients enrolled in the system. For example, if the more costly of two therapeutic alternatives is associated with a lower hospital readmission rate, use of the more expensive product might be well justified.

The potential for pharmacist leadership on important health system issues is just beginning to be explored. New insights are expected to emerge at a conference ASHP is conducting on pharmacy in integrated health care systems in July 1995. Among the topics that will be discussed are pharmacy issues that influence the success of an integrated health care system, population-based approaches to establishing drug use policies, options for providing pharmaceutical care to ambulatory patients, and innovative partnerships with the pharmaceutical industry. ASHP has also increased the focus on outcomes management and pharmacoeconomics in its educational programming.

It was the clear emergence of integrated systems that led ASHP to change its name from the American Society of Hospital Pharmacists to the American Society of Health-System Pharmacists (3). This change was approved by ASHP members in a mail ballot in the summer of 1994 by a three-to-one margin. At the time, 13% of the society's practitioner members were based in components of health systems other than hospitals, including home health care and HMO ambulatory care clinics. We expect that this percentage will grow substantially in the years ahead.

Although ASHP's recent name change struck some observers as a precipitate action, it had been in the works for nearly 20 years. In 1975, reflecting emerging trends in the hospital field, ASHP changed its purview from hospital pharmacy to pharmacy in "organized health-care settings." At the time, it was noted that hospitals were often at the center of a multifaceted health care system and that the principles that had guided hospital pharmacy practice were frequently applied in other forms of organized health care delivery. Those observations of two decades ago still ring true today.

## *HOSPITAL REENGINEERING*

While the hospital field's big-picture people are developing integrated systems, hospital operational managers are trying to make their institutions work better. One observer recently summarized this development by commenting that hospital administrators have come to recognize:

> that cost reimbursement fostered haphazard and inefficient operations. There was a tendency to create new patient services as islands, squeezing the latest one among the others, with confidence that the money would be there to cover the cost. Services were developed primarily from the hospital worker's perspective, not the patient's. Adjusting this perspective is the goal of patient-focused care, a movement that continues to build momentum and has already had a major impact on the hospital industry. (4)

A consultant who advises hospitals on reengineering their operations made these observations:

Perhaps one of the triumphs of the hospital industry has been to convince patients and physicians that they are getting decent service. What they get, by and large, is incredibly lousy service. Turnaround times for routine items, initial medication orders, routine x-rays, and routine laboratory work can only be described as excessive. (5)

Hospital management's answer to this serious problem has been to change the structure of hospital operations. The goal is to build operations around the needs of patients, not the convenience of hospital departments. Often, departmental workers such as pharmacists and pharmacy technicians are redeployed to individual patient care teams. Work simplification, cross training of personnel, decentralization of services, interdisciplinary collaboration, use of treatment protocols, elimination of layers of management, and increased involvement of patients in their own care are among the tools used to achieve restructuring (6). With the aid of consulting firms, reengineering along the line of patient-focused care concepts is a common occurrence. ASHP data show that patient-focused care has been implemented in more than 22% of hospitals with 200 or more beds; it is under development or consideration in more than 44% of hospitals of that size (1).

Patient-focused care certainly has merit, but we have worried that if it is carried to an extreme, it could be detrimental to the wise use of pharmaceuticals in hospitals. We believe that the pharmacy department in a hospital must have sufficient status to permit leadership in the following areas:

1. Fostering optimal use of pharmaceuticals
2. Achieving effective cost control of pharmaceuticals
3. Improving the institution's overall competitiveness
4. Transforming pharmacy into a patient-focused profession. (7)

Consistent with their interest in reengineering, hospital managers are making big investments in computerization and automation. Illustrative is the latest ASHP survey in which 89% of hospitals had a computerized medication information system, up from 75% in 1992 and 64% in 1990 (1). Of those hospitals not computerized, nearly half said they had approval to obtain a computer system within the next year. Similarly, there is significant interest in automating hospital drug distribution. For example, 20% of nonfederal hospitals use decentralized drug dispensing units (i.e., automated vending machines), and another 14% plan to begin using them within the next year (1).

These trends in computerization and automated drug distribution, combined with substantial use of pharmacy technicians, support a shift in the pharmacist workforce from drug product handling to drug therapy management. ASHP data indicate that increases continue to occur in the extent to which hospital pharmacists offer services such as written drug therapy management plans for individual patients, drug therapy monitoring, educating or counseling patients, and written medication histories (1).

## THE COMPOSITE HOSPITAL PICTURE

Both the macrolevel and microlevel changes in hospitals are responses to the current national policy of reducing the use of expensive acute care (inpatient) services and shifting more patient care to subacute care, long-term care, home care, and ambulatory care settings. The acute care portion of hospital operations has been shrinking. Between 1983 and 1993, the number of inpatient days among community hospitals declined 21%. The number of community hospitals in that period fell 9% (8). Within the past year, the number of inpatient days declined 2.6% (9). On the other hand, hospital outpatient visits were up 75% over the decade ending in 1993 (8). For the most recent year, the number of hospital outpatient visits went up 6.3% (9).

We anticipate that many pharmacists employed in acute care will be shifting their focus to home care and ambulatory care. Quite often, they will be able to make these career moves without switching employers as their hospitals become integrated with larger delivery systems.

## PHARMACEUTICAL CARE

Pharmacy practitioners in all sectors of practice are in the process of shifting their mission from drug dispensing or distribution to pharmaceutical care, a practice concept that puts the pharmacist in a position to help individuals achieve optimum outcomes from medication use (10). Two imperatives have caused pharmacy practice to move in this direction: (1) societal need for an expert in safe, effective, and cost-conscious use of medications and (2) pharmacists' self-interest in the preservation of their profession.

Within hospitals and health systems, there has been strong interest in pharmaceutical care. ASHP sponsored a conference in 1993–the "San Antonio conference"–that outlined practitioner strategies for transforming pharmacy practice along the lines of this model (11). At the heart of the recommendations that came out of San Antonio is the idea that the staff of each pharmacy department should go through a consensus-building process on the need to transform practice in this manner and to map out a systematic strategy for bringing about this change.

For ASHP's part, it launched a rich array of programs designed to help foster the implementation of pharmaceutical care. For example, the ASHP Foundation has funded a series of state and regional conferences, patterned after the San Antonio program, that led practitioners to explore the basic truths of the concept and how it may be put into practice. The society has created the Clinical Skills Program, a program designed for use in staff development with the aim of giving practitioners the skills they need to provide pharmaceutical care. Overall, ASHP's publications and educational programming focus on how practitioners can transform their practices in ways that will position pharmacists to help people make the best use of medications.

Similar efforts are occurring professionwide. For example, the 1994 Pharmacy in the 21st Century conference, which was sponsored by the Joint Commission of Pharmacy Practitioners (JCPP), concentrated on implementation issues for all areas of practice. (JCPP is a federation of national pharmacist practitioner organizations.)

Although hospital pharmacists have become strong believers in the need to reengineer their profession, it is difficult to change the fabric of their practice because the pharmacy department does not exist in a vacuum; it is buffeted by others' expectations and stereotypes of pharmacists. In the most recent ASHP national survey of hospital pharmacy departments, about 47% indicated that pharmaceutical care is provided to some extent to their patients. However, only 8% covered more than half of their patients (1). Even though changing to a pharmaceutical care focus is a very difficult task, practitioners recognize that there is little choice but to move in this direction if they want to survive as a health profession.

## IMPLICATIONS FOR PHARMACEUTICAL MARKETING

Given the three megatrends discussed above–the development of integrated health care systems, hospital reengineering, and pharmaceutical care–what will a smart pharmaceutical marketer do to prepare for success in this new environment? We would not presume to prescribe the specific course of action for any company, but we do believe that seven ways of thinking about the market will be the keys to success (12).

*The Target Market.* Recognize that the target market is not hospitals but integrated health care systems that provide a continuity of care to patients in all settings, including acute care. For the near term, integrated systems may still segregate pharmaceutical purchases for their inpatient populations, but they will begin deciding what to buy in terms of which products will achieve the best patient outcome.

*The Purchasing Function.* Recognize that the functions of some organizations involved in institutional drug purchasing will be assumed by integrated health care systems directly. For example, group purchasing will probably be taken over by many integrated systems. Likewise, some systems will take on the pharmacy benefit management function for ambulatory patients.

*Formularies.* Recognize that formularies and formulary management will still be relevant concepts but their underpinning will be systemwide pharmacoeconomics, not acquisition cost and not solely an inpatient perspective. Pharmacists will continue to play a key role in formulary development and management as they learn how to be guided by pharmacoeconomic and outcomes data.

*Ambulatory Patients.* Recognize that hospitals will sometimes be the base for an integrated system's pharmaceutical services to ambulatory patients. Fifty-five percent of hospital pharmacy directors expect that their departments will devote more attention to ambulatory care in the future (1).

*Virtual Inventory.* Recognize that there will be growing interest in just-in-time delivery of pharmaceuticals (especially for expensive products) for all components of integrated health care systems, including acute care, home care, long-term care, and ambulatory care. In the acute care setting, these deliveries may short-circuit the central pharmacy and go directly to the patient care areas of the hospital. Under such arrangements, it will still be important for health system pharmacists to review initial medication orders and to manage the overall drug use process. A related development will be growth in off-site preparation of IV admixtures and other compounded dosage forms for use in acute care and home care. Drug wholesalers will probably play an important role in this development, which suggests that there is a need to explore three-way joint ventures by an integrated system, a drug manufacturer, and a drug wholesaler.

*Disease State Management.* Recognize that this topic, all the rage today among leading pharmaceutical manufacturers, is probably relatively short-lived as an industry function. As integrated health care systems mature and grow in sophistication, particularly in their development of advanced information systems, they will learn that the best way to manage diseases is to empower their health professionals with the necessary information and the authority to do the job, taking into account the specific needs and desires of individual patients.

*Pharmaceutical Care.* Recognize that the goals of pharmaceutical care are consistent with the interests of the pharmaceutical industry. Fundamentally, it is to a drug company's advantage if the decisions about the use of its products are tailored to the needs of individual patients. That is the goal of pharmaceutical care; centralized, cost-driven edicts about the use of pharmaceuticals work against the idea of the pharmacist taking responsibility for the optimum outcome of medication use. Hence, the efforts of pharmacy practitioners to transform their profession merit the understanding and support of the pharmaceutical industry.

## CONCLUSION

Just as the hospital industry and pharmacy practice in institutional settings are going through significant changes, so will the marketing of pharmaceuticals to hospitals change greatly. This is not a negative factor; it is simply the reality of the market-driven reforms unfolding in institutional health care. Behind these changes is the hope that the new order will result in more cost-efficient care without compromising the humane, respectful, and science-based treatment that patients desire and deserve. We all should be working toward that goal.

## REFERENCES

1. Santell JP. ASHP national survey of hospital-based pharmaceutical services–1994. Am J Health-Syst Pharm 1995;52:1179-98.

2. Shortell SM, Gillies RR, Anderson DA. New world of managed care: creating organized delivery systems. Health Aff 1994;13:46-64.

3. Anon. Answers to 10 common questions about ASHP's name change. Am J Health-Syst Pharm 1995:52:75-6.

4. Zellmer WA. Leadership priorities for 1995. Am J Health-Syst Pharm 1995;52:224.

5. Lathrop JP. Patient-focused care from the consultant's viewpoint: we didn't plan it this way. Am J Health-Syst Pharm 1995;52:45-8.

6. Vogel DP. Patient-focused care. Am J Hosp Pharm 1993;50:2321-9.

7. Zellmer WA. Advice to hospital executives: elevate the pharmacy. Am J Hosp Pharm 1993;50:2450.

8. AHA. Hospital statistics–the AHA profile of United States hospitals, 1994-95 edition. Chicago: American Hospital Association, 1994.

9. Anon. Key trends through third quarter 1994. AHA Econ Trends 1995;10(4):11.

10. Hepler CD, Strand LM. Opportunities and responsibilities in pharmaceutical care. Am J Hosp Pharm 1990;47:533-43.

11. Anon. Implementing pharmaceutical care: proceedings of an invitational conference conducted by the American Society of Hospital Pharmacists and the ASHP Research and Education Foundation. Am J Hosp Pharm 1993;50:1585-656.

12. Zellmer WA. Rethinking hospital pharmaceutical marketing. Am J Health-Syst Pharm 1995;52:1590.

# Marketing to Managed Care Pharmacy: Think Local, Think Partnerships, Think Outcomes, Think Disease State Management

William Tindall

## LESSONS OF MANAGED CARE FOR THE PHARMACEUTICAL INDUSTRY

The year 1994 was one in which it would have been very difficult to find someone who did not believe that America's health care system needed reforming and who did not support health reform out of fear and compassion. Some feared they might lose their health insurance because of lack of portability or not get it because of preexisting conditions; others supported universal access to health care as a right, especially for the uninsured. Later in 1994, the political stir for health care reform subsided when polls showed that 83% of all insured were content with the quality of their health care and that for Mr. and Mrs. America, crime, the economy, and jobs were higher on the list of concerns. In addition, other polls indicated that 93% of Americans did not want government selecting their physicians, and they further believed health insurance was an obligation of their employers. As a result, in 1995, health care reform is not stirring the political fervor it once caused, although there is movement toward allow-

William Tindall, Ph.D., is Executive Director of the Academy of Managed Care Pharmacy, 1321 Duke Street, Suite 305, Alexandria, VA 22314.

[Haworth co-indexing entry note]: "Marketing to Managed Care Pharmacy: Think Local, Think Partnerships, Think Outcomes, Think Disease State Management." Tindall, William. Co-published simultaneously in *Journal of Pharmaceutical Marketing & Management* (Pharmaceutical Products Press, an imprint of The Haworth Press, Inc.) Vol. 10, No. 2/3, 1996, pp. 177-193; and: *Pharmaceutical Marketing in the 21st Century* (ed: Mickey C. Smith) Pharmaceutical Products Press, an imprint of The Haworth Press, Inc., 1996, pp. 177-193. Single or multiple copies of this article are available from The Haworth Document Delivery Service [1-800-342-9678, 9:00 a.m. - 5:00 p.m. (EST)].

ing states to experiment with reform through Medicaid and Medicare waivers, tort and insurance reform, and new ERISA interpretations. These developments mean that 1995 will be a year in which payers, providers, consumers, and purchasers of health care will continue to be drawn to managed care for its ability to reduce health expenditures while preserving quality. Also in 1995, states will attempt to reform their health insurance acts, medical malpractice acts, health planning processes, provider availability, scope of professional practice, and the pharmaceutical industry's pricing system. Some of these attempts are misguided and anticompetitive to managed care. But managed care is finding that anticompetitive legislative measures bring new alliances with consumer groups (as happy patients), some state governments (as public purchasers), and some employer groups (as private purchasers) of managed care. While many Americans hoped in 1994 that the federal government would do something about health care costs and access, the health care system has continued down the long road to reform encouraged by favorable marketplace conditions and the Health Maintenance Organization Act of 1973. As more and more Americans enroll in managed health care, five observations can be made. These observations are important to a manufacturer of pharmaceuticals and to any other vendor of health goods and services trying to compete in a system transforming from indemnity or fee-for-service funding to managed care funding (Figure 1):

1. Managed care changed health care at a rapid pace while bringing increased competitiveness, documented savings, and improved quality.[1]
2. Managed care is growing in acceptance by Americans, and it is here to stay.
3. As more people accept managed care as patients, providers, or payers, they relate to each other more positively.
4. Managed health care is like politics (very local), so if you want to deliver safe, effective, timely health care offering value for the dollar, then effective relationships are needed at the local level.
5. Managed care relationships are built on a new paradigm of value wherein health care is defined as a service and patients, payers, and providers are empowered as customers.

## THE PHARMACEUTICAL MANUFACTURER IN AN ERA OF CHANGING RELATIONSHIPS

Managed care, by simple definition, is a unique American business practice. It is founded on relationships that are mostly *quid pro quo* and

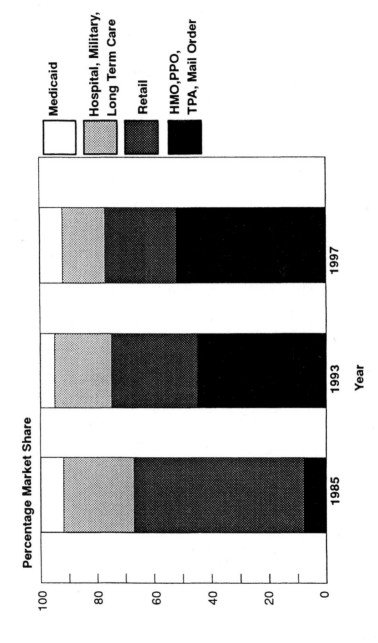

FIGURE 1. Growth in Pharmaceutical Sales 1985-1997.

hold accountable appropriate care to patients, outcomes, and cost-effectiveness. But because managed care redefines relationships on the basis of providers, patients, and payers being customers of each other, pharmaceutical manufacturers have to rethink who their customers really are. Today's pharmaceutical customer is no longer the solo practice physician who for nearly a century has been targeted with messages about a drug's safety, efficacy, and therapeutic equivalency. Rather, the pharmaceutical industry's customer has become the decision maker(s) within a managed care organization (MCO) or a pharmacy benefit management company (PBM) (Figure 2). These decision makers are growing daily and so is their sophistication in local/regional markets where they command market share or volume purchasing through leveraging economies of scale.

A pharmaceutical manufacturer whose marketing staff has long used direct mail, journal ads, samples, and detailing is finding that these are not targeted messages reaching decision makers in managed care. To reach the managed care customer, the pharmaceutical manufacturer must first build a relationship based on mutual understanding of each party's needs. Manufacturers must also be alert to rapidly changing market conditions and cannot rely on economic models that have stood for decades, such as price inelasticity in the demand for drugs. Instead, today's manufacturer is

FIGURE 2.   What Motivates New and Traditional Buyers of Pharmaceuticals.

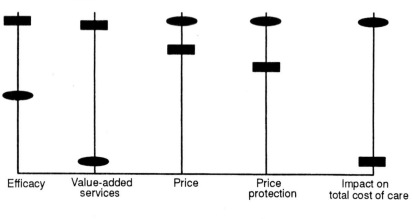

Source: Deloitte & Touche LLP, Management Consulting 1995

a player in a new ball game where not-so-clearly-understood rules are being used, such as the demand for outcomes research, disease state management services, pharmacoeconomic data, and other tools used to sharpen the ability of a managed care organization to deliver value for the dollar.

Because of the need for trusting relationships and new marketing messages, pharmaceutical manufacturers have three simple ways to respond to the new marketplace reality of managed care: learn to ignore it, change it, or change themselves. Because it is easier to change themselves, drug manufacturers have initiated three simple strategies. The first is to win new business from managed care organizations, whose formulary management systems favor generics (a number of brand-name manufacturers have bought, borrowed, or begged alliances/buyouts with generic firms). As a marketing strategy, this enables the brand-name manufacturer to place off-patent products into competitive positions with volume discounting. The second strategy involves the manufacturer getting into the disease state management business by either buying a pharmacy benefit management company or starting one of its own (Table 1). Today at least 15 disease management programs have been started, many of them product based.

TABLE 1. New Examples of Vertical Integration for Disease State Management.

| Drug Manufacturer | | Disease State Management Company |
|---|---|---|
| Bristol Myers Squib | joined | Caremark |
| Caremark | invested in | Technology Assessment Group (TAG) |
| Eli Lilly | bought | Integrated Disease Management/PCS |
| Merck | bought | Medco Containment Services |
| SmithKline Beecham | bought | Diversified Pharmaceutical Service |
| Pfizer Inc. | joined | Value Health Inc. |
| Upjohn | started | Greenstone Healthcare Solutions |
| Zeneca | started | Stuart Disease Management Service |
| Zeneca | bought | Salick Health Care |

A third strategy has been corporate reorganization through reengineering, downsizing, right sizing, or applying some populist corporate philosophy to meet the needs of managed care. For example, many pharmaceutical manufacturers have reengineered their pharmaceutical representative into a new national account manager or NAM. This NAM has essentially one performance measurement tied to his or her job–get the company's products on as many formularies as possible. This may not be too difficult if the NAM has developed a strong working relationship with the managed care decision maker(s) in his or her territory and can understand a managed care organization's needs for his or her products. As managed care markets become more localized, the opportunity exists for a local NAM to deal with local decision makers to meet each other's needs. Interestingly, for some time the NAM is likely to be an enigma within his or her own company as traditional marketers continue their marketing plans–which push safety, efficacy, equivalency, and price–while failing to understand that the NAM operates in a world where a managed care decision maker may ask for product guarantees, risk contracts, or proof that a product actually lowers overall health care costs while contributing to the patient's quality of life. In a market where one or two managed care entities dominate, getting the NAM's products on one or two formularies is paramount to building and retaining market share and very often his or her job. Very often, the NAM's decision maker is the director of pharmacy for an HMO, PPO, indemnity insurance company, or a PBM, a person not traditionally seen as a customer and who has become very empowered. A director of pharmacy in a managed care setting takes on new significance as a customer when the pharmacy and therapeutics committee staffed by that pharmacist provides pharmaceutical care for 1,000,000 patients or more per year. Inclusion in managed care formularies will become increasingly important for pharmaceutical manufacturers, and to obtain a formulary listing they will need to move into the realm of disease state management and outcomes research. In summary, the NAM will have to think of local conditions, think on his feet, think creatively, and think selflessly. A good start for the pharmaceutical manufacturer's NAM would be to ask himself or herself the following three questions:

1. Am I here to satisfy myself or my customers?

2. If the answer is my customers, what are their needs?

3. What could I be doing better to meet those needs?

# PHARMACEUTICAL MARKETING, PHARMACEUTICAL CARE, AND OUTCOMES RESEARCH

To managed care pharmacists, pharmaceutical care is well defined and can be implemented with admirable success and savings using the skillful application of ten special tools (Tables 2 and 3). These tools rely on: (1) outcomes-based formularies, (2) guidelines and protocols that encourage prescribers, pharmacists, and patients to adhere to "appropriate drug use," and (3) management information systems or databases that, when analyzed, provide patient information showing how costs per member per month (PMPM), length of stay (LOS), quality of life years (QOLY), or some other measurable outcome is affected by pharmaceutical care and benefit design. Interestingly, these same pharmacists are quick to point out that measurable outcomes in a pharmacoeconomic study done in Boston do not necessarily transfer to a managed care organization in Omaha, Nebraska. This is because as managed care pharmacy directors' knowledge about pharmacoeconomic studies has increased, they have become more discerning. They are pretty much aware that each managed care site has different patient databases, different economies of scale, different costs of doing business, different demographics, and different diseases being treated; thus, they insist on doing more of their own tailor-made local studies. Even though many pharmaceutical manufacturers fund pharmacoeconomic studies where the medical and pharmacy databases can be integrated, there is a benefit for both the MCO and the manufacturer if they work together. The manufacturer can use information from a pharmacoeconomic study to enhance its ability to demonstrate a product's cost-effectiveness while that same study may give the MCO feedback on the value of its pharmaceutical care interventions. Regardless, both the

TABLE 2. Savings Offered by Prescription Benefit Plans.

| | |
|---|---|
| Clinical Programs | up to 15% |
| Bids and Contracts | up to 17% |
| On-line Adjudication | up to 3% |
| Audits | up to 3% |
| TOTAL | up to 38% |

Source: Academy of Managed Care Pharmacy, 1995

TABLE 3. Ten Tools to Build a Prescription Benefit Under Managed Care Concepts.

| Tool | Useful For |
|---|---|
| 1. Pharmacy and Therapeutics Committee | a) choosing safe and effective drugs |
| | b) setting in place formulary management |
| 2.. Therapeutic Equivalency Programs | a) choosing best product |
| 3. Generic Equivalency Programs | a) allowing manufacturers, bioequivalency, and bioavailability factors to interplay. |
| | b) providing incentives for patients through differential copays |
| 4. Bids and Contracts | a) capitalizing on economies of scale |
| 5. Academic Detailing | a) educating prescribers to use appropriate therapy protocols |
| 6. Coinsurance | a) shifting budgets to patient |
| 7. Dispensing Limitations | a) reducing waste and sharing of drugs |
| 8. Drug Utilization Review (DUR) | a) evaluating patients compliance |
| 9. Drug Utilization Evaluation (DUE) | a) evaluating physician's prescribing habits |
| 10. Outcomes Management | a) evaluating medication on a cost-effective basis and impact on quality of life |

Source: Academy of Managed Care Pharmacy

manufacturer and the MCO must be sure that the study withstands scrutiny, as there is still a lot of skepticism about the credibility of this type of joint research because of its considerable variation from well-understood clinical trials (Table 4).

Pharmaceutical company executives are faced with a difficult dilemma in assigning corporate resources to traditional clinical trials versus the long, expensive, large sample size pharmacoeconomic studies. They trust either expense will be offset by having their product included in a managed care formulary after having spent up to two years doing these studies.

TABLE 4. Pharmacoeconomics: What the Techniques Mean.

Cost-Benefit Analysis (CBA)–This method compares the costs and benefits of treatment alternatives in terms of dollars. It requires converting benefits, or outcomes, into dollar values. This may be difficult with some benefits, such as years of life saved.

Cost-Effectiveness Analysis (CEA)–Similar to CBA but does not require converting outcomes into monetary units. Instead, costs of treatments being compared are related to the same outcome nonmonetary units, such as cost per years of life saved.

Cost-Minimization Analysis (CMA)–Used to compare costs if two or more treatments have been shown to be equally effective in similar patients. Outcomes, being equal, are not measured. CMA is used when comparing costs of different dosage forms of one drug or generically equivalent drugs that have been shown to be equally effective.

Cost-Utility Analysis (CUA)–Examines costs of treatments in relationship to the costs of their outcomes, for example, the cost to treat side effects or the cost of neonatal intensive care in a premature infant. These costs are then evaluated in terms of the treatment's impact on the patient's quality of life, for example years of life gained. The value of a state of health to the patients studied is determined by a survey of a random sample of the general population who rank the outcome of the treatment.

Source: C.E. Reeder, Managed Care Pharmacy Practice, Dec. 1994

Another caveat is that pharmacoeconomic research may not prove that a drug product is more cost-effective than a "me-too" drug. However, outcomes research is growing and is the justification for about one-third of the formulary decisions made today. Those in managed care who believe in outcomes-based formularies need pharmacoeconomic information that probably could not have been obtained without a partner. Likewise, when partnered appropriately, pharmacoeconomic information gives the manufacturer the chance to have information on how its drug is used in the real world.

## PHARMACEUTICAL MARKETING
## AND DISEASE STATE MANAGEMENT

The next logical step for any pharmaceutical manufacturer that wants to get close to its managed care customer, has committed to conducting outcomes research, and has formed an alliance or integrated with a pharmacy benefit management company is to climb on the bandwagon of disease state management (Table 5).

The objective of disease state management is to offer a managed care customer team-driven protocols and interventions and the capability of monitoring for specific costly diseases for which the manufacturer has the appropriate pharmaceutical products and the requisite background of expertise. This let-me-give-you-a-helping-hand approach is being viewed somewhat gingerly by those in managed care pharmacy who believe it runs counter to the concept of treating the whole patient in an integrated system of care, in spite of the manufacturers' good intentions and counter-balancing point of view (Figure 2)(Table 6).

Despite some skepticism surrounding disease state management, it is being implemented not only by pharmaceutical houses and PBMs but also by some managed care organizations; using their own initiatives (Figure 3). An example is Group Health Cooperative of Puget Sound, a mixed-model HMO of nearly 400,000 members, which has introduced to its members its "Clinical Roadmap" program. Group Health offers systematic disease management initiatives that focus on managing care rendered to

### TABLE 5. Disease State Management Defined.

Disease state management is a comprehensive and integrated health care provider/plan strategy that leads to more effectively and efficiently preventing and treating specific disease states. It involves the patient, the health care provider, and the entire health care system.

Source: Marion Merrell Dow

### TABLE 6. Marion Merrell Dow's Point of View on Disease State Management.

- ○ Disease state management is not a quick fix nor an overnight solution to decrease cost;

- ○ It is not a new marketing strategy;

- ○ Disease state management strategies are a provider/health care system/plan issue;

- ○ Marion Merrell Dow has competencies to help identify and meet customer emerging needs;

- ○ Disease state management is redefining our business.

FIGURE 3.The Functions of Disease State Management.

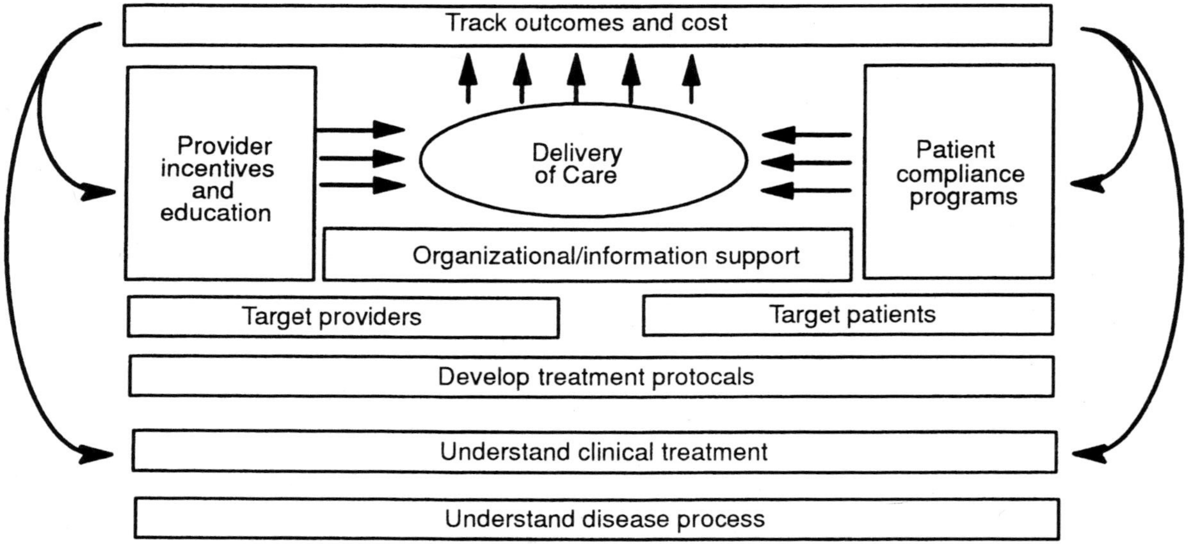

Source: Health Industries Research Company

187

specific patients, but it does so by adjusting the Group Health delivery system to facilitate the best outcome.

A recent example of a pharmaceutical manufacturer's innovative approach to disease state management is the purchase of Salick Health Care by Zeneca. Salick lends value to Zeneca, for it is a major service provider of cancer care. As a result, Zeneca has access to medical records that it could not obtain through other means. While Salick's strength is its carve-out arrangement with managed care organizations, issues such as confidentiality of patient records and conflict of interest were fears that were easily resolved when Zeneca declared that its practice guidelines would be made public.

Despite trepidation and obstacles, more and more managed care organizations are developing disease management programs, with partners (e.g., the Pilgrim Health Care-Glaxo Asthma Program) or without them (e.g., Intermountain Health Care, the Mayo Clinic) (Figure 4). Diseases getting the most attention are asthma, AIDS, cancer, cardiovascular disease, depression, diabetes, hypertension, and pneumonia because they exhibit the criteria most amenable for a disease state management program, i.e., they are chronic diseases with cost components much greater than pharmaceuticals, and there has been a move to formularies that list only two or three drugs within a therapeutic area (Table 7).

The average length of time an employer stays with a single carrier is a little under two years, causing some to question the existence of the incentive to conduct long-term pharmacoeconomic studies to assess disease management programs. Still, it does appear that disease state management programs will grow and that pharmaceutical manufacturers will partner with managed care organizations to make them happen. These partnerships will require the pharmaceutical manufacturers to approach the managed care organization in entirely new and open ways, otherwise the MCO is likely to close the manufacturers out, do the programs anyway, and call its new findings proprietary. Once a pharmaceutical manufacturer and an MCO join together on a disease state management program, there must be a clear understanding of critical success factors before the program is initiated. These critical success factors must be responded to first if credible outcomes research is to be conducted.

Pharmaceutical manufacturers will see disease state management continue to grow. This growth will be fueled by the growing realization that treatment costs for chronic conditions consume a larger portion of the health care dollar. Growth will also continue because sophisticated research of integrated managed care databases will permit pharmaceuticals to be purchased and pharmaceutical care to be delivered on the basis of

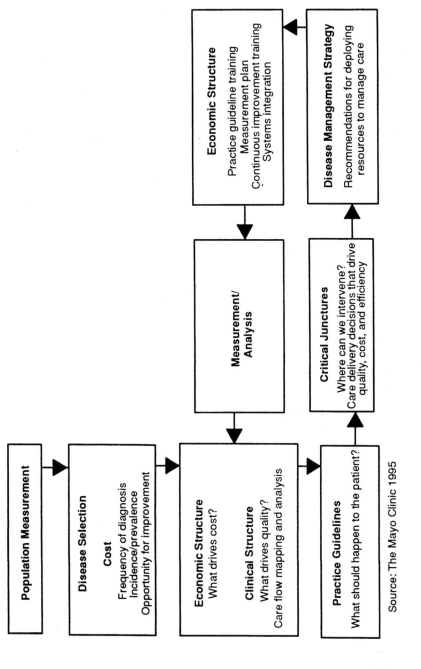

FIGURE 4. The Mayo Clinic's Disease Management Strategy.

**Population Measurement**

**Disease Selection**

**Cost**

Frequency of diagnosis
Incidence/prevalence
Opportunity for improvement

**Economic Structure**
What drives cost?

**Clinical Structure**
What drives quality?
Care flow mapping and analysis

**Practice Guidelines**
What should happen to the patient?

**Measurement/ Analysis**

**Economic Structure**

Practice guideline training
Measurement plan
Continuous improvement training
Systems integration

**Critical Junctures**

Where can we intervene?
Care delivery decisions that drive
quality, cost, and efficiency

**Disease Management Strategy**

Recommendations for deploying
resources to manage care

Source: The Mayo Clinic 1995

TABLE 7. Seven Criteria That Make a Disease Suitable for Disease State Management.

1. The disease has a high incidence of preventable emergency room and other hospital treatment.
2. The disease has a high incidence of inappropriate prescribing and patient noncompliance.
3. The disease affects a large population.
4. The disease creates high costs visible to an employer.
5. The disease lends itself to improvement via patient education.
6. The disease treatment lends itself to timely, measurable, outcomes.
7. The disease is chronic and requires long-term managment.

rational value-driven decisions (Table 8). As the new discipline of disease state management evolves, one can expect it to run on a continuum from a disease-focused product marketing approach whose goal is drug utilization to its more appropriate goal of managing outcomes, which is more extensive and expensive and relies on quality of life measurement. Either way, there will be plenty of work for the pharmaceutical marketer in changing the behavior of prescriber, patients, and pharmacists.

## THE PHARMACEUTICAL MARKETER AND THE NEAR FUTURE

The pharmaceutical marketer or NAM who recognizes that managed care's formulary management, practice guidelines, outcomes research, and disease state management can fundamentally shift the manner by which his or her employer will make a profit through their impact on the research-intensive pharmaceutical industry's product life cycles will do well. As the industrialization of American health care continues, it makes good sense for pharmaceutical manufacturers to continue to forge win-win relationships with their managed care customers and to base those relationships on a mutual understanding of each others' therapeutic and economic contributions. There is an emerging trend that will facilitate those relationships and provide new marketing opportunities. That trend is the growth of integrated health systems (IHS) in America, as well as in Europe (Figure 5). Health systems in Europe may be very different from

TABLE 8. Questions Necessary for a Disease State Management Program.

1. Are there existing appropriate treatment protocols that can save **time** and money?

2. Are there well-defined patient outcomes that need improving?

3. Are the patient outcomes measurable?

4. Is there a plan to integrate all appropriate therapies in order to study them?

5. Is there a plan to deal with comorbidities?

6. Is there a plan to reimburse or compensate for the disease state management service?

7. Will the program allow caregivers to perform at their best?

those in the U.S., but they face the same problems of escalating costs and a growing elderly population.

During the last half of the 1990s, managed care's market dominance with HMOs, PPOs, indemnity insurance, and PBMs is reengineering to introduce a full spectrum of health care delivered through an integrated network or integrated health care system. The response to this reengineering is a rapid growth in mergers, acquisitions, and alliances between hospitals, physicians, insurers, health plans, MCOs, and related providers. This integration of health care is seen as a response to four conditions driving the consolidation of the local health care purchasing system: (1) financial drivers, which influence the shape of contracts with payers and providers, (2) physician hospital drivers, which link patient referrals, (3) clinical drivers, which influence patient access and the continuum and coordination of care, and (4) information drivers, which support the other three drivers.

How an integrated health system is built depends a lot on local market conditions and demographics. For example, a health system in Minneapolis is quite different from one in Tampa. For that reason, pharmaceutical manufacturers like Marion Merrell Dow, Merck, Glaxo, and others have split their marketing departments into well-defined managed care and IHS regions. This gives them an opportunity to get close to their customers and the influence these customers have on drug distribution. During the last half of the 1990s, it makes good marketing sense to view integrated health systems, which could have upwards of 400,000 patients and 1,500 doctors, as customers through which a pharmaceutical manufacturer could "channel" its drug products.

The Health Industry Research Company (HIRC) expects that the 14 million people currently enrolled in 70 integrated health systems at the start of 1995 will grow to 52 million people enrolled in 220 IHSs by the

FIGURE 5. Managed Care vs. Integrated Health Care.

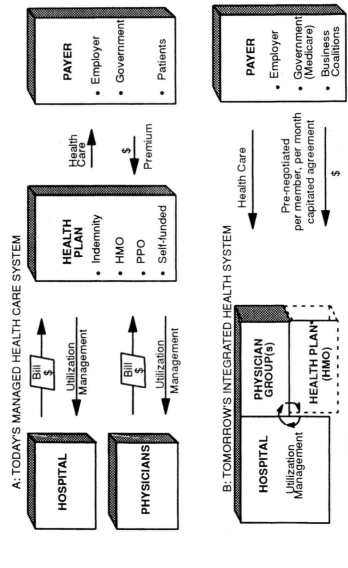

A: TODAY'S MANAGED HEALTH CARE SYSTEM

B: TOMORROW'S INTEGRATED HEALTH SYSTEM

*May be owned or closely affiliated.
**Health Industries Research Company**

year 2000. Intermountain Health Care in Salt Lake City and Henry Ford Health System in Detroit are two good examples of integrated health systems. For integrated health systems to keep market share, they must pay attention to five interlocking systems: materials management, systems development, utilization management, operations, and patient satisfaction. For the pharmaceutical marketer who understands these systems, opportunities to build relationships and service will continue as they have in managed care. One may also predict that as integration among health care providers continues there will be supportive roles for pharmaceutical companies to help with marketing, actuarial, financial planning, risk taking, and other joint ventures.

## THE BOTTOM LINE

The pharmaceutical industry and managed care organizations will continue to share common concerns. These concerns range from patient outcomes to rising costs to political initiatives such as unitary pricing and ERISA waivers. Such concerns lead both to demand successful partnerships. Before each enters a partnership, however, it will assess the other's needs, research capabilities, formulary control, and communication channels to form an honest, open, trusting (H.O.T.) partnership that leads to a win-win outcome. Once these partnerships are in place, the partners will position each other as essential members of a local health care team. Both will find that their partnership yields a good return on investment if their marketing messages focus on outcomes (i.e., pharmaceutical products + cost-effectiveness data + managed pharmaceutical care = outcomes offering value for the health care dollar) and project an appreciation for the contributions of each to those outcomes.

## NOTE

1. The Congressional Budget Office (CBO) and the American Managed Care and Review Association Foundation estimate savings of 12.6% to 13.6%.

# Pharmaceutical Marketing
# in Lesser Developed Countries

## Albert I. Wertheimer

### INTRODUCTION

Pharmaceutical marketing in lesser developed countries cannot be easily fit into a one-size-fits-all description, unfortunately. However, there are a number of common features. Before we embark on this journey of marketing practices exploration, it is appropriate that we define some terms. For the purposes of this review, let us look at the world in three levels of development, or categories (1).

First, we have the areas of North America, the U.K., Western Europe, Japan, Australia, New Zealand, and some other isolated examples, such as Iceland, Israel, and South Africa, among others, that we can refer to as developed (2). Next, there are perhaps 20 nations that may best be described as developing. Examples include Taiwan, Malaysia, Indonesia, Egypt, South Korea, and perhaps Brazil, Argentina, India, and Hungary, to mention some examples. These developing nations have, in many cases, a complete and well-developed industrial base and infrastructure, educated skilled workers, and usually a stable economic system (3).

The third category is the least developed countries. Many are quite poor and have very limited industrial resources. Most of the population works in agriculture and has little or no formal education. Many of these nations lack public health services; higher education; and telephone and highway

Albert I. Wertheimer, Ph.D., is Vice President for Pharmacy/Managed Care at First Health Services Corporation, 4300 Cox Road, Glen Allen, VA 23060.

[Haworth co-indexing entry note]: "Pharmaceutical Marketing in Lesser Developed Countries." Wertheimer, Albert I. Co-published simultaneously in *Journal of Pharmaceutical Marketing & Management* (Pharmaceutical Products Press, an imprint of The Haworth Press, Inc.) Vol. 10, No. 2/3, 1996, pp. 195-205; and: *Pharmaceutical Marketing in the 21st Century* (ed: Mickey C. Smith) Pharmaceutical Products Press, an imprint of The Haworth Press, Inc., 1996, pp. 195-205. Single or multiple copies of this article are available from The Haworth Document Delivery Service [1-800-342-9678, 9:00 a.m. - 5:00 p.m. (EST)].

systems that are stable, reliable, and functional. Some lack very basic sanitation, water supply, food and medicine distribution, and even rural electrification. The majority of examples here are found in Africa, Asia, and to a lesser extent, in Central and South America.

What adds to the confusion is the fact that most of the developing and least developed countries have combinations of (1) wealthy, educated persons who are members of privileged families owning and/or controlling natural resource assets such as mines, forests, and plantations or owning local industries and (2) peasants who are individuals and families who work in agriculture, if at all. The presence of a robust middle class is generally missing in the least developed countries. A middle class is growing in the developing countries and is being filled with middle management, technical persons, and those in the conventional professions (4).

## UNDERSTANDING THE SITUATION

This spectrum of income and wealth is important for our analysis. The reason for this bifurcation is that a nation having an upper class and a lower class has two separate and distinct health care delivery systems, and they must be viewed individually. One of the features shared by the lesser (least) developed countries is that the vast majority of the population depends upon the state for the provision of personal health services. The large cities, including the national capital and provincial capitals, generally have hospitals, and attached to them are outpatient clinics. Smaller towns may have a health post or dispensary, and rural villages may have traveling health care providers who visit the village a few days each month–when the roads permit–or a nurse or semi-trained health worker residing there on a permanent basis. Often, this latter category, when it exists, is little more than a small one-person first-aid post. What was just described may be referred to as the public sector health system (5).

Public sector patients receive services and drugs at little or no fee in most cases. It is common to wait half a day or longer to see a service provider at such crowded clinics, and drug use is limited to what is available at the clinic. There is some probability that the drug will be out of stock or that the supplies present might have passed the expiration date. Therefore, the closest therapeutic equivalent will be dispensed. We will return to the management of drug supply in the public sector later.

### PRIVATE SECTOR

In the private sector, the scene is not unlike what residents of Western nations experience. One visits a private physician, or a physician who sees private and public patients, to eliminate long waits. The physician writes a prescription, and the patient takes it to a community pharmacy where it is dispensed in a typical private commercial transaction. Sometimes prices are fixed, and in other cases, the health authorities have no control over a purely private transaction. The prescribed drug is quite likely to be the same product that the large, multinational firms are currently selling and promoting in the U.S., the U.K., or France. Well, then, one might ask, what are the rules and policies governing private sector promotion, marketing, and advertising? This is an easy question to ask, but a difficult one to answer, in general, as there are probably as many answers as there are lesser developed countries (6).

Many of the lesser developed countries received independence from previous colonial powers within the last 30 years, and their priorities have been basic infrastructure issues such as defense; police; supply of foods; finance and taxation; highways; water supply; sewage; and production of domestically educated technicians, engineers, and physicians. What this means in practical terms is that there may be no food and drug law, or it may be the one inherited from the previous colonial nation, or there may be legislation that is ineffective, or there may be realistic legislation but no funds to enforce or police it. In all of these scenarios, there is little protection for the public or assurance for the physician that the drugs on the market are safe and efficacious.

As a typical strategy to avoid risk, it is commonplace for physicians practicing in the private sector environment to write prescriptions for branded products from large and well-respected Western European or North American based firms. In this way, all but counterfeited products and unauthorized generic substitution risk can be eliminated. Drug marketing regulations in the least developed countries, as a rule, are minimal and usually unenforceable (7).

## MARKETING PRACTICES

The incentives and behaviors are quite easy to understand and to appreciate. The prescriber knows of countless examples of misbranded or adulterated generic drugs, counterfeit drugs, and products sold well past their expiration dates. Therefore, he orders well-known, popular branded products, hoping to have the security that the patient will receive what was ordered. In addition, manufacturers' representatives visit physicians to detail the latest outstanding medications that are being used by physicians in New York, Bonn, London, and Paris. A certain comfort level is achieved by the physician. Also, the physician is ordering a drug that is clearly unattainable through the public sector, another reason patients pay a fee to consult with this physician. Generic drugs dispensed through the public sector rarely have a wholesale cost of more than $5 to $10 per 100 tablets, whereas a branded product might have a wholesale cost of $30 for 30 tablets (8). Perhaps the assumption is that a drug this costly must be good or that persons who can afford to visit a private practice physician can surely afford the imported branded product or would want a product available only to the elite of that society.

Many of the least developed countries have no FDA and no means of policing marketing regulations. It is thought that the worst abuses in claims for indications and in downplaying of side effects come from local manufacturers and not from the multinational companies. Sales representatives from manufacturers visit physicians to inform them of top-selling products in the major cities in Western Europe and North America. Why shouldn't this physician's patients have access to the same miracle drugs enjoyed by others around the world?

Where potential problems arise here is with the information presented to the prescriber. In most developed countries, the FDA or its equivalent agency specifies what indications may be mentioned and what prescribing cautions, interactions, side effects, and warnings must be included in any promotional messages. However, in some lesser developed countries, there is often minimal–or no–mention of cautions or warnings, and the indications may well be a bit expanded from what is considered acceptable in the developed West (9).

## *CONSUMER PROTECTION*

It would not be fair to say that all of the examples of inappropriate promotional activities continue today, as the industry has made great strides to police itself. In fact, the International Federation of Pharmaceutical Manufacturers Associations (IFPMA) has published a voluntary Code of Pharmaceutical Marketing Practices. This is clearly a big step in the right direction. The limitations to this project include its voluntary status, the inability of the IFPMA to get tough with its members, and the fact that perhaps only about 20% of the worldwide pharmaceutical industry organizations are members of the IFPMA. Most smaller domestic firms operating exclusively in lesser developed countries are not IFPMA members (10).

Assisting in the campaign to rein in pharmaceutical marketing practices that seem to be excessive or less than 100% honest and/or incomplete with regard to side effects, cautions, and warnings are several international consumer protection and advocacy groups. One is Health Action International (HAI), which is most active in Europe. The International Federation of Consumer Unions, located in Penang, Malaysia, and Medlam from Australia actively work to counteract less-than-candid drug promotion. This work is similarly performed on some occasions by Social Audit in London and by Public Citizen's Health Research Group in Washington, D.C.

The job of regulating pharmaceutical marketing is extremely difficult. Just imagine the full extent of the work necessary to catch verbal messages of an illegal content even though the printed matter is in compliance with international standards. Such a Herculean task would require countless hours of agency time and perhaps still result in failure to catch any wrongdoers. Some countries require changes in labeling, package inserts, and changed or new promotional material to be approved or cleared in advance by an agency within the Ministry of Health. Knowledgeable persons tell of having to wait two or more years for authorization for such submissions. The other approach, as exemplified by the United States practice, is to put the responsibility for accurate, evenhanded, and complete information upon the shoulders of the manufacturer. The drug company can use promotional messages as it sees fit, but should a message be found to be misleading or incomplete, the FDA has the authority to order the company to cease and desist from the offending practice. The FDA can then require the firm to distribute remedial messages to physicians and pharmacists or face substantial financial penalties (11).

Having explained these approaches in theory, it is nothing less than honest to indicate that in the former case the company often goes ahead without receiving an official authorization after 6 or 9 or 12 months have passed without any government reply. Manufacturers may feel secure about doing this when they realize that hundreds of other companies are in the same situation. In the second scenario, there are abuses found also. Many people appear to know that the drug control agency is underfunded and understaffed and that perhaps only the egregious violations will be pursued by the authorities.

Again, it is not possible to make broad, sweeping generalizations, but there appears to be some level of acknowledgement by industry veterans that gifts, favors, and other considerations for agency civil servants can protect a firm from criticism or can ensure that the inspectors will be looking in the other direction when a likely violation may be undertaken in some countries.

There is every reason to believe that the World Health Organization (WHO) will continue to work in concert with the International Pharmaceutical Federation (IPF), HAI, the World Council of Churches, and other agencies, in addition to the IFPMA, to improve marketing practices of pharmaceutical producers and distributors throughout the world in the coming years (12).

## CONSUMER BEHAVIOR

In a separate but related issue, the reality is that in many countries within the lesser developed world, prescription drugs are distributed rather differently from what is considered routine in the West. It is commonly the case that a patient enters a private pharmacy shop and describes a problem or symptom to the shop clerk (or pharmacist, should the latter party happen to be present). The clerk will then sell a product—which could be an antimalarial, antibiotic, muscle relaxant, or whatever—to the patron without the benefit of a doctor's diagnosis or prescription (13).

The incentives for this behavioral sequence are strong and real on both sides of the dyad. For the client, going directly to the pharmacy saves perhaps a one-day wait at a clinic or a significant fee if a private physician were to have been consulted. There would have always been the possibility that, after the public clinic visit, the individual would have had to visit the pharmacy anyway if the clinic did not have the desired drug in stock. For the pharmacist, there is the satisfaction of helping a fellow citizen obtain needed drug therapy at a reasonable price and certainly on a more timely basis than through the alternative scenarios.

Many of the medical journals commonly found in the West—*JAMA, New England Journal of Medicine, Lancet, Medical Letter*—often do not reach such areas, so pharmacists and physicians are forced to depend on manufacturer-supplied "educational" materials (14).

The Letters to the Editor sections of medical and pharmacy journals throughout the world, especially during the 1970s and into the 1980s, were full of reports of marketing problems in lesser developed countries. Some of those receiving the most attention included promotion of vitamins with anabolic steroids for slow-growing children, chloramphenicol for upper respiratory diseases, steroids for a host of conditions, and antibiotics for trivial infections probably caused by viruses. Fortunately, one sees fewer and fewer letters calling attention to such undesirable practices today.

## MARKET CHARACTERISTICS

Changing the subject slightly, it should now be apparent to the reader that there is little potential reward or payoff for drug manufacturers to undertake promotion in the public sector. The public sectors in lesser developed countries have learned how to accumulate their orders to obtain favorable quantity prices and how to send out tenders requesting bids from generic drug manufacturers. Ministries of Health may do this directly to a list of qualified bidders around the world, or they may choose to turn this chore over to a local or international firm that would seek bids from potential suppliers and negotiate on behalf of the Ministry for the best terms. Or the Ministry may elect to order directly from UNIPAC, the supply arm of UNICEF, in Copenhagen. This supply operation purchases drugs from around the world at incredibly inexpensive prices, tests them, and repacks them into various sizes of bottles and tin drums. Hard currency paid at the time the order is placed is required. Most of the drugs are from generic sources (15).

Some countries choose to prepare their own drugs for the public sector. Some of this involves basic synthesis, such as in Indonesia and in the Philippines. Other countries purchase bulk intermediates and prepare the final dosage forms. Public sector clinics and other facilities normally use a formulary list which shows a physician which drugs are prescribable. Nearly all of these are multisource items following the patent expiration of the originator products.

By contrast, real marketing opportunities exist in the private sector. Recall that it is customary for patients to request a drug for a condition, and usually, they do not request a drug by its trade name. Therefore, pharmacies purchase products having high profit margins from those available through branded sources. There are detail people in virtually all countries of the world, and these representatives inform physicians about new products and about new uses for older products. Samples and token gifts are often left in the physician's office (16, 17).

In many lesser developed countries, personal selling is the principal form of marketing and sales promotion. The postal services are often unreliable, and there are not occasions such as symposia and continuing education sessions held on a regular basis, or even frequently. The value of the medical service representative is immense in such countries. In many of these countries, there is no medical or pharmaceutical journal published on a regular basis, and where journals are published, they tend to devote more attention to association news and gossip than to scientific or professional features. This lack of a journal denies an advertising vehicle to manufacturers and slows down the dissemination of new scientific information to practitioners, again increasing the importance of the representatives.

## *DISTRIBUTION*

Distribution is important in and of itself, but it is even more critical in lesser developed countries. If a product is out of stock, practitioners will use an alternate, and should they like its efficacy, they might switch to the alternate product as their preferred drug in that category. Distribution is handled in several ways. One is for a multinational firm to have an office for a region in a capital city that is responsible for 2 or 3 or even 5 or 6 adjacent countries. Often, the inventory is kept at that one depot, although it is possible for supplies to be kept at the homes of each of the representatives. In this way, representatives not only make a sale but actually deliver the goods and complete the transaction.

In addition to the locating of a sales force, supply depots, etc., another option is to name a local company as an agent. The manufacturer ships inventory to its agents, and the sales reps for this agent visit physicians and pharmacists, take orders, deliver the merchandise, collect payment, and perform other marketing and representational duties.

A third alternative is for a manufacturer to have no formal or direct presence but to sell to wholesalers and other distributors who either use or resell the products. In this third model, there is no real, or even implied, continuing relationship as seen in the second model. In fact, in the second model, often the agent also handles regulatory activities and governmental and professional interfaces, advertising, public relations, and the like. In all three options, the field force is almost always comprised of local persons who, of course, know the language, customs, and political/economic infrastructure. Not only can they intelligently (usually) discuss the product, but they can also chat comfortably about local sports and politics (18).

Personal selling is of monumental importance in any case, and the allocation of resources to this function is similar to what is seen in developed countries. The well-known and respected professors at the teaching hospitals, who by nature of their positions become opinion leaders, are targeted for intensive sales promotion activities, as might be expected. The goal of marketers is to have these opinion leaders become loyal prescribers of specific products. In accomplishing this, countless future medical students will be exposed to the product as the one (indirectly, at least) recommended by this respected academic medical leader.

## *REGRETTABLE NOTES*

This section is not intended to pass judgment, but the essay would be incomplete if this component were missing. It is axiomatic that there is a great deal of poverty in many lesser developed countries. Also, many hardworking and dedicated civil servants, health care providers, and other workers professionals and nonprofessionals alike–lead a precarious existence. Some government workers are owed their salaries for fairly long periods of time, creating a difficult situation for them and their families. This situation is compounded by the fact that civil servants and those working for the government routinely earn substandard wages. Sometimes, the temptation is too great to resist when a little gift can be obtained simply by specifying one brand over another. The extent of said practices varies by region, individual, and country and by the current economic situation. It is said that in some places one can get a drug approved, get a drug approved more rapidly, get a drug on a formulary, or have a favorable price fixed by providing money to the other party. If these are common practices participated in by all, one can try to rationalize the behavior as the norm in that country. However, someone eventually pays for the gifts and favors.

Franchises, licenses, protected distributorships, judgeships, and other important political appointments are sometimes made in consideration for favors and contributions to the ruling party or to government officials. Let us hope that such practices are on the decline and that greater democracy, a more educated population, less poverty, a robust middle class, and the development of consumerism and public interest advocacy groups can stem the tide of the less desirable features mentioned here.

## SUMMARY AND CONCLUSIONS

Marketing, no matter where it takes place, independent of country, language, wealth, or even planet, must provide the famous "4 P's." There are just more challenges and barriers in some places than in others. The challenges to successful pharmaceutical marketing are overwhelming in numerous lesser developed countries. Even the most adroit salesman or marketer can do little when reckless government fiscal policies permit massive inflation rates, when bribery is condoned, when foreign exchange is simply unavailable to be used to pay for imported goods, when the telephones fail to operate, or when the roads are impassable in rainy seasons. No matter how skilled a salesperson may be, he or she cannot overcome Ministry of Health paralysis on approvals or labeling changes, shortages of gasoline, shortages of automobile parts, electricity rationing, curfews, violence, tribal battles, petty crime, government delays in clearing customs paperwork, tardy ordering practices, and probably hundreds of other routine events in lesser developed countries (19).

To be sure, it remains the duty of a marketer to educate and to create demand for a product. Quite amazingly, that is what is being done in even the most remote and isolated hamlets of the world by dedicated professionals doing the best that they can, considering the obstacles facing them.

Perhaps a stint in such an environment would be splendid training for domestic marketers. As a personal note and epilogue, it seems only reasonable that the firms that deal with lesser developed countries today with respect and integrity will have a major advantage in those countries that pull themselves up and have real purchasing power 10 or 15 years from now. Support of educational offerings; donations of reference books and textbooks; and responsiveness to professional, government, and academic inquiries and requests should pay off handsomely in the future when those countries generate the ability to return favors and pay debts (20).

## REFERENCES

1. Anon. Formulation of comprehensive national drug policies, DAP. Geneva: World Health Organization, May 1981.

2. Schneider M, Dennerlein RK, Kose A, Scholtes L. Health care in the E.C. member states. Amsterdam: Elsevier, 1992.

3. Basch PF. Textbook of international health. New York: Oxford University Press, 1990.

4. Anon. Health conditions in the Americas. 1990 ed. Vol. 1, nr. 524. Washington, DC: Pan American Health Organization, 1990.

5. Tucker D. The world health market. New York: Facts on File Publications, 1984.

6. Roemer MI. National health systems of the world. Vol. 2. New York: Oxford University Press, 1993.

7. Spivey RN, Wertheimer AI, Rucker TD. International pharmaceutical services. Binghamton, NY: Pharmaceutical Products Press, 1991.

8. Lapatra JW. Healthcare delivery systems evaluation criteria. Springfield, IL: C. C. Thomas Publishers, 1975.

9. Adenika FB. Pharmacy practice management in developing communities. Lagos, Nigeria: Literamed Ltd., 1985.

10. Kanji N, Hardon A, Harneijer JW, Mamdani M, Walt G. Drug policy in developing countries. London: Zed Books, 1992.

11. Burrell CD, ed. Drug assessment in ferment: multinational comparisons. Washington, DC: Interdisciplinary Communication Associates, 1976.

12. Anon. World health statistics annual, 1985. Geneva: World Health Organization, 1985.

13. Anon. Drug labeling in developing countries. Washington, DC: Office of Technology Assessment, February 1993.

14. Quick JD. Managing drug supply. Boston: Management Sciences for Health, 1981.

15. Anon. International health statistics. Washington, DC: Office of Technology Assessment, 1993.

16. Anon. The use of essential drugs. Technical report series, nr. 722. Geneva: World Health Organization, 1985.

17. Anon. World Health Organization Expert Committee on Specifications for Pharmaceutical Preparations: 27th report. Geneva: World Health Organization, 1980.

18. Anon. National drug policies, public health in Europe. Vol. 12. Copenhagen: World Health Organization Regional Office for Europe, 1977.

19. Reich, MR, Eiji M. International cooperation for health. Dover, MA: Auburn House, 1989.

20. Spector RE. Cultural diversity in health and illness. New York: Appleton Century Crofts, 1979.

# Trends in Drug Distribution Channels and Practices

Bruce R. Siecker

## *WHOLESALE DRUG DISTRIBUTION TODAY*

As America prepared to eat its evening meal and settle down to homework, watch television, and play PC games last night, an amazing thing was happening between the nation's pharmacies and their ever-ready drug wholesalers. More than 100,000 different orders totaling more than 1 million items were making their way through the vast maze of telephone, fiber-optic, and microwave channels to seek out electronic listening posts that are maintained by the country's full-service, full-line drug wholesalers.

By the time most people were asleep, drug wholesalers were hard at work. Orders that arrived electronically, some as recently as an hour before, were interpreted by the drug wholesaler's computer, and inventory levels in primary storage-picking areas were checked by the computer. If necessary to process a night's orders, sufficient inventory was moved from secondary to primary storage positions, where actual order filling is done. The order fulfillment process had begun–quietly, accurately, and efficiently.

Late into the night, wholesale drug warehouse workers gathered each item for each order from numerous storage areas that house 18,000 to 28,000 different and distinct items within highly secured warehouses. One million individual items were retrieved from open stock-picking areas;

Bruce R. Siecker, Ph.D., is President of Business Research Services, Inc., 12713 Franklin Farm Road, Herndon, VA 22071-1914.

[Haworth co-indexing entry note]: "Trends in Drug Distribution Channels and Practices." Siecker, Bruce R. Co-published simultaneously in *Journal of Pharmaceutical Marketing & Management* (Pharmaceutical Products Press, an imprint of The Haworth Press, Inc.) Vol. 10, No. 4, 1996, pp. 207-221; and: *Pharmaceutical Marketing in the 21st Century* (ed: Mickey C. Smith) Pharmaceutical Products Press, an imprint of The Haworth Press, Inc., 1996, pp. 207-221. Single or multiple copies of this article are available from The Haworth Document Delivery Service [1-800-342-9678, 9:00 a.m. - 5:00 p.m. (EST)].

items ordered in full cases were pulled from case storage. Some inventory items were gathered manually. Other items were picked from semiautomated systems, where machines and people combined to make the process extremely efficient and accurate. In still other cases, totally automated picking systems selected and assembled pharmacy orders at speeds that must be seen to be appreciated.

Some items were wrapped in protective materials to prevent damage; others were picked and stored cool, cold, or frozen if necessary. Controlled substances were signed out very carefully from caged areas and high-security vaults. Some personnel handled products that must be accompanied by Material Safety Data Sheets, while other distribution center personnel prepared trip-route schedules and customized pharmacy shelf labels and price stickers for every item being sent according to each pharmacy's unique pricing policies. Wholesaler systems are so sophisticated today that they are even smart enough to print extra price stickers to be used on stock already at the pharmacy when there has been a price increase since the last time a pharmacy ordered a particular item.

At the end of what can appear to be mass confusion to the untrained eye, different parts of an individual pharmacy's daily order began to merge in a final sorting and staging area. Orders were assembled, checked, and then loaded into vehicles. To make the delivery process the most efficient possible, each pharmacy's order was loaded into a vehicle by delivery route and in reverse delivery order. By as early as 5:00 a.m., orders began their journey to each pharmacy, often arriving as or before the pharmacy was opening for the day or by midday at the latest.

All of this occurs every night, 5 to 6 days a week, 52 weeks a year. In addition, there are instances where a drug wholesaler makes more than one delivery a day or delivers emergency needs. The pharmacy resupply process is transparent to everyone outside the industry, as millions of bytes of electronic intelligence find their way to each wholesaler's computer, and it is accomplished with amazing accuracy and efficiency.

Drug wholesalers enable every pharmacy in America, no matter how small or remote, to purchase inventory in the right amount and at the right time. Drug wholesalers also provide numerous valuable adjunct services to their customers for much less than these services are available elsewhere. What is especially amazing about this modern drug distribution marvel is that the overall costs to the pharmacy are lower than any other form of distribution. Today's wholesale drug distribution system is unmatched anywhere in the world in terms of its performance and contributions to the health and economic well-being of this country.

## MARKETPLACE, MARKET SHARE, REVENUE DYNAMICS

Drug wholesalers generated $47.5 billion of economic activity in 1993, which was 11.5% more than in 1992. The figure for 1994 may easily top $51 billion. Sales growth for drug wholesalers has been steady and impressive in the past eight years, as seen in Table 1.

As revenues have continued to grow, so has the drug wholesaler's market share. Full-service, full-line drug wholesalers now account for 80% of all pharmaceuticals distribution in the U.S. The reasons for this growth are many, but drug wholesalers continue to enjoy a large market share primarily because they provide an accurate, reliable, efficient, low-cost set of services. In addition, their customers prefer the prime vendor resupply channel over other forms of distribution. Drug wholesalers have also been pursuing an effective market-share strategy that is supported by continuously shaving margins and prices as a result of operating efficiencies.

What drug wholesalers are selling, to whom they are selling, how much they are charging for their services, what margins are generated from operations, what it costs to produce those services, and what–if anything–is left over at the end of the year have continued to evolve. As is evident in Table 2, today's drug wholesalers are primarily distributors of pharmaceuticals. Although the percentage of pharmaceutical sales to total sales is essentially static, sales growth in dollars is substantial.

Nonprescription drugs continue to be the second largest product category. Nonprescription drug sales are growing in dollar terms, though declining as a percentage of total sales. Health and beauty aids (HBA), the third largest category, are growing in importance in total dollars and as a percentage of total sales. These 3 categories accounted for more than 93% of a typical drug wholesaler's sales mix in 1993, and there are few indications that this concentration will change materially in the near future.

While product mix is relatively stable, with the exception of the nonprescription drug and health and beauty aid categories, and weighted heavily toward pharmaceuticals, the drug wholesaler's customer base is evolving along a number of fronts (Table 3). Independent drugstores sales have declined in the past two years as a percentage of sales, although dollar sales are still increasing. Chain drugstore sales have been fluctuating, and no clear trend is evident.

The sales figures appear to indicate that chain warehouses have virtually disappeared as a customer group. In the strict sense of sales from wholesaler inventories, this is an accurate depiction, but it does not tell the whole story. Drug wholesalers also do what are called nonstock sales, where they buy from suppliers on behalf of customers (almost as a broker,

TABLE 1. Total Industry Sales in Billions of Dollars and Percentage Change from Previous Year, 1986-93.

| 1986 | 1987 | 1988 | 1989 | 1990 | 1991 | 1992 | 1993 |
|---|---|---|---|---|---|---|---|
| $16.3 | $19.5 | $22.2 | $25.2 | $30.2 | $36.2 | $42.0 | $47.5 |
| 18.5% | 16.8% | 14.0% | 13.5% | 18.2% | 15.2% | 17.0% | 11.5% |

Source: The NWDA Operating Survey, 1993

TABLE 2. Percentage Sales by Product Type, 1989-93.

|  | 1989 | 1990 | 1991 | 1992 | 1993 |
|---|---|---|---|---|---|
| Rx Drugs | 80.6% | 79.5% | 79.2% | 81.7% | 80.7% |
| Non-Rx Drugs | 8.4 | 10.0 | 11.5 | 10.1 | 9.7 |
| HBA | 6.7 | 7.1 | 6.6 | 5.4 | 6.8 |
| Gen. Merchandise | 2.2 | 1.9 | 1.2 | 1.4 | 1.6 |
| DME/HHC* | 1.0 | 0.9 | 1.1 | 0.9 | 0.8 |
| Other | 0.9 | 0.6 | 0.6 | 0.5 | 0.4 |

* Durable medical equipment and home health care
Source: NWDA Operating Survey, 1993

but different in that they actually take title to the goods) and then immediately transship (called "across the dock" or "cross dock" sales) the orders to those customers. This business segment is growing substantially and more than offsets the apparent disappearance of the chain warehouse as a viable customer in these figures.

The preponderant growth category in terms of increasing market share is sales to hospitals, which moved from 23.9% of sales in 1989 to 29.0% in 1993. Although still one of the smaller categories, sales to grocery and mass merchandisers is growing impressively in both dollar and share terms, 2.8% to 6.0% in only 5 years, or $707 million to $2,322 million from 1989 through 1993.

## *CONSOLIDATION AND SCALE ECONOMIES*

Drug wholesalers continue to react to changes in the marketplace and evolve to meet its demands. The industry has consolidated dramatically in

TABLE 3. Drug Wholesaler Sales by Type of Customer, 1989-93.

|  | 1989 | 1990 | 1991 | 1992 | 1993 |
|---|---|---|---|---|---|
| Independents | 40.9% | 40.8% | 41.4% | 39.1% | 36.7% |
| Chain Drugstores | 22.2 | 25.7 | 23.5 | 22.0 | 22.7 |
| Hospitals | 23.9 | 22.9 | 26.7 | 27.1 | 29.0 |
| Chain Warehouses | 7.5* | 2.8 | 1.1 | 2.0 | 0.1 |
| Grocery & Mass Merchandisers | 2.8 | 4.3 | 3.2 | 4.9 | 6.0 |
| Clinics & Nursing Homes | 1.2 | 1.0 | 2.5 | 2.6 | 3.1 |
| Others | 1.6 | 2.5 | 1.6 | 2.3 | 2.4 |

* Prior to 1990 chain warehouse sales were reported inconsistently. Figures from 1990 forward are consistent and reliable.
Source: NWDA Operating Survey, 1993

the past ten years. In 1983, there were more than 150 different drug wholesale companies serving the 50 states. Today the number is approaching 50, and there are predictions of fewer than 20 different companies by the turn of the century.

With consolidation and growing sales, drug wholesalers have continued to build much larger distribution centers. In 1983, the average drug wholesaler warehouse did less than $30 million in sales each year; the same figure for 1993 was $173 million. There were approximately 375 warehouses in 1983, fewer than 250 in 1993. Some of the newer megacenters are more than 250,000 square feet and are capable of handling a billion dollars or more of business a year. Larger distribution centers have allowed drug wholesalers to continue to take advantage of dramatic advances in automatic identification, material handling, and information processing technologies.

Prevailing wisdom in the industry, which is generally supported by industry performance statistics, is that bigger is better in designing distribution centers. Drug wholesalers have augmented larger designs with creative and cost-effective use of bar-coding technologies, automated storage and picking systems, and state-of-the-art information processing. With the possible exception of mail-order pharmacies, no part of the drug industry even begins to match the drug wholesaler's sophisticated use of technology.

## FALLING PRICES AND MARGINS BY DESIGN

All of these efforts have allowed drug wholesalers to garner a larger market share by continually lowering their prices. Some prices are so low that pharmacies can often buy products from drug wholesalers for less than they would pay if they purchased the products directly from the manufacturer. The availability of lower prices and an essential array of value-added services that a pharmacy would not get from a drug manufacturer helps explain why the drug wholesaler is so popular.

Drug wholesalers have dramatically and continuously reduced the cost of drug distribution and have reduced the cost of health care by tens of billions of dollars. As one industry leader stated at the 1994 annual meeting of the National Wholesale Druggists' Association (NWDA) in addressing health care reform, "the administration could have used the wholesale drug industry as a case study in selling its ideas on health-care reform. The wholesale drug industry has returned billions of dollars to the U.S. marketplace. . . . "

Lower prices–especially when gross margins are already the thinnest in history–work only so long as they produce enough new sales to offset lost margin dollars that result from lowering prices. Drug wholesaler pricing strategies have indeed produced increased sales and increased market share; they have also depressed operating margins. To counter the impact of price reductions, drug wholesalers have managed to continue to reduce operating costs as a percentage of sales. Lower prices have driven up sales; scale economies and the creative and intensive use of technology are reducing costs. The combination, *at least so far,* has been enough to keep drug wholesalers reasonably profitable in an increasingly tough marketplace.

As Figure 1 demonstrates, drug wholesaler margins have (with several exception years) continued to drift downward. Figure 1 reports gross margin. It is important to recognize that gross margin is not the same as markup. A drug wholesaler's gross margin is an amalgam of markup, shrinkage, damaged goods, prompt payment discounts, financial leverage, and forward buying. At the same time, operating expense reductions have offset most (if not all) of the decline in operating income (income from operations before tax) that would have resulted from a continuing decline in gross margin. The top line represents average gross margin by reporting year for full-service, full-line drug wholesalers. An overall gross margin for 1984 of 9.74% declined almost 4 percentage points by 1993 to 5.82%. This represents a 40% decline in gross margin percentage. The bottom line in Figure 1 represents operating income. It is arguable whether operating

FIGURE 1. Drug Wholesalers' Gross Margins, Operating Expenses, and Profit, 1984-1993.

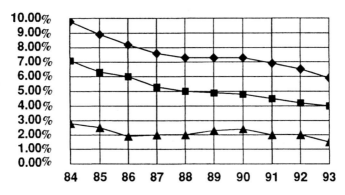

Source: NWDA Operating Survey, 1993

income is actually trending downward, but what began as 2.90% for 1983 ended the 10-year span at 1.78%, or about 1.1 percentage points lower.

The reason that operating income did not fall four percentage points is explained by the operating expense line (the middle line in Figure 1). Drug wholesalers were able to reduce operating expenses by almost three percentage points during the same decade. This major accomplishment allowed drug wholesalers to avoid about three-fourths of the negative effects of declining margins on their profitability, which in turn made it much easier to offset lower prices with the margin from increased sales.

## THE THREE-CYCLE "DOOMSDAY" ENGINE

During the second half of the 1980s, drug wholesalers accelerated their bid for increased market share. In doing so, they became even more competitive and ever more willing to cut prices (and therefore margins) in an effort to attract business. The underlying assumption of this strategy was that increased sales from new sources–in essence, making the pie bigger rather than relying solely on taking business from another wholesaler–will more than offset lost margin dollars as a result of cutting prices.

Lower prices attracted more new business, which drug wholesalers competed for by lowering their prices even more. The only ways to keep pace were (a) to find ways to cut operating expenses still further and (b) to take advantage of the buying profits that drug manufacturers were offering as a result of their rapid escalation in prices.

Drug wholesalers have historically invested heavily in updating their distribution centers and in finding ways to use more efficient mechanical and electronic technologies. Efforts aimed at handling products and information more efficiently do reduce operating costs, and drug wholesalers pursued such efficiencies with zeal during the second half of the 1980s.

During this era, drug wholesalers were generating significant gross margin from three sources: markups on goods sold to their customers, cash discounts for prompt payments to suppliers, and forward-buying profits as a result of manufacturers' price increases. According to at least one analyst, the smallest contribution to gross margin during this period was from buying and selling products, while forward buying accounted for upwards of 75% of some drug wholesalers' gross margins.

## PARADIGM SHIFTING BY CHOICE

It was generally apparent to drug wholesalers that operating costs could not reach zero, and so, by definition, their market-share strategy was finite. (The unspoken goal was that 100% distribution could be achieved before margins and expenses crashed into the horizontal axis.) As margins continued to inch lower, drug wholesalers began to ponder their next move. What was missing was a way to stop the three-cycle "doomsday" engine that was driving drug wholesaling. Greater operating efficiencies were lowering costs; lower costs allowed still lower prices. Smaller markups attracted still more business. More business, in turn, helped reduce costs still further as a percentage of sales. But so long as drug prices continued to escalate rapidly, there was no doomsday. Drug wholesalers continued to fuel their growth, reinvestment, and profit requirements through buying profits, and there was little to stop the process.

The risk of these strategies over the long term was driven home to drug wholesalers, however, when drug prices stopped inflating so rapidly at the beginning of the new decade. When that happened during the second half of 1992, a major source of gross profit virtually disappeared, and the industry's profits began to suffer. Wholesalers found themselves with very large, very efficient drug distribution centers–some estimate the industry had and still has as much as 40% overcapacity in its aggregate physical plant–but with less business left to capture (because their market share was already high) and extremely thin operating margins.

During this period, there were several industry-level and individual initiatives aimed at forging new industry partnerships (little "p") as a way of redefining "the business" and derailing the runaway three-cycle engine. A concomitant purpose was to give drug wholesalers an opportunity to increase the size of their marketplace, to take advantage of innovative thinking in interorganizational information systems, and to explore new services wholesalers might perform for (and hence be paid for by) their suppliers.

The National Wholesale Druggists' Association, through its "breakthrough" initiative, led efforts to open up military, public health, and VA depot markets to drug wholesalers' prime vendor programs. NWDA spearheaded a historic effort to create a highly efficient electronic information system called HEALTHCOM® and supported and nurtured partnering trials between pairs and groups of drug wholesalers and manufacturers.

## THE HEALTH CARE REFORM JUGGERNAUT

Just as these so-called "breakthrough" initiatives were beginning to address the economic realities of slower drug price inflation and its effects on the market-share strategy, the drug industry was shaken to its core by the specter of health care reform that was spawned by the November 1992 Presidential elections. The attention paid to health care reform triggered changes in drug industry thinking, attitudes, and behavior that are so far beyond anything the industry has ever witnessed that there is simply no historical benchmark by which to assess it. The drug industry had survived, virtually untouched, all manner of disruption in the past, including the elimination of fair trade laws in the 1950s, the Medicare and Medicaid Acts of 1965, the advent of diagnosis related groups reimbursement in 1983, and more recently, Medicaid rebates. But now, long-term industry thinking and practices were fundamentally and irreversibly changed *without any federal legislation ever being passed.*

The health care reform debate also set off a flurry of activity in drug wholesaling. It dramatically rekindled a consolidation and buyout frenzy that continues even today. Most partnering experiments that only months before had shown substantive promise withered or were abandoned altogether. Drug manufacturers soon began talking quite differently. They talked gravely about how each company in each segment of the distribution channel now needed to look out for itself. At the same time, they started buying each other and pharmacy benefit management companies. Many began massive restructuring programs–initially described as "downsizing," later changed to the wonderful euphemism "right sizing"– in a frantic attempt to reverse decades of marketing and staffing practices in time to be able to weather and survive whatever might come out of Washington as a result of health care reform. According to at least one report, there are more than 38,000 fewer people employed by pharmaceutical manufacturers than before the brouhaha of health care reform.

The national health care reform debate by itself (actually, there have been a number of changes to state laws and programs that are real and did and do require attention) caused the drug industry to engage in a massive program of self-administered financial surgery and operational liposuction. The industry's reaction to the health care reform debate has been dramatic and substantive. It reacted in extreme ways and to such an extent that it will never again be the way it was prior to 1993.

There are enough announcements in the press about new buyouts, mergers, sell-offs, and other signs even today to suggest that industry consolidation and restructuring has not run its course. There are those (the writer included) who believe that it has yet to peak and that the drug industry will emerge from this period as a much different species.

## RISE OF SPECIALTY DRUG WHOLESALING

With little fanfare and limited attention (until recently), a new type of drug wholesaler is emerging. Similar to what were once called limited-line or short-line wholesalers (meaning that they did not stock and sell a wide range of product lines), specialty wholesalers are differentiated by the *types of products* that they distribute or the *types of customers* to whom they distribute.

The major types of specialty wholesalers in the market today limit their product lines to what are loosely termed specialties, e.g., biologicals, parenterals, biotech drugs, and/or oncology drugs. Their niche often includes selling to types of customers that full-line, full-service drug wholesalers have yet to begin servicing or have chosen not to service. In some cases, drug manufacturers are using specialty drug wholesalers because of the wholesalers' ability and willingness to collect and report certain types of information or the fact that the wholesalers do not carry competing lines of products.

Specialty drug wholesalers are an interesting dynamic for two reasons. First, drug manufacturers have, up to this time, generally treated specialty drug wholesalers as a separate class of trade. The rationale for doing so appears to center around the wholesalers' willingness and ability to service customer groups that a drug manufacturer needs to address (and which are not addressed by full-service, full-line drug wholesalers) and the different types of services that some specialty drug wholesalers provide. As a separate class of trade, specialty wholesalers are able to purchase at materially lower prices in spite of the fact that they sometimes compete directly with mainline drug wholesalers. Second, at least so far, specialty wholesalers have not shown any willingness to give away what in effect are extra margins by lowering their prices. This tends to indicate a marketing strategy that favors differentiation rather than a low-price, market-share approach.

To date there is little, if any, systematic information, other than anecdotal, on the size and scope of specialty drug wholesalers. Given the paucity of information, very little can be said with confidence about trends in specialty drug wholesaling and whether such entities will continue to specialize or are bound by "business DNA" to evolve into full-service, full-line distributors. If and when specialty drug wholesalers form their own trade organization or join with their larger counterparts as members of the NWDA, more will be known about this segment of drug distribution.

## DISTILLING THE DRUG WHOLESALER ROLE

Setting aside market specifics, it is useful to consider what roles a drug wholesaler plays in the drug distribution channel and how these roles are valued today. To some people, a drug wholesaler is simply a "middleman." As a middleman, these people believe, a drug wholesaler does nothing more than add cost to the system. This impression is shortsighted, inadequate, and completely wrong!

Drug wholesalers in the pharmaceutical industry are merchant wholesalers, which means that they purchase, take title, and pay for goods they buy from drug makers and marketers. In doing so, drug wholesalers act as customers for, investors in, and storers of a manufacturer's products. Typically, a drug wholesaler will buy pharmaceuticals frequently from 75 to 100 major manufacturers and less frequently from several hundred smaller suppliers.

Without drug wholesalers, each of the several hundred pharmaceutical producers would have to establish, maintain, and service upwards of 60,000 to 80,000 different pharmacy, hospital, clinic, government, and others types of accounts. Many of those accounts–probably up to half–would order infrequently, in relatively small quantities, and be slower payers. Because of distances, shipping times, and order minimums, pharmacies would have to stock significantly more inventory. Pharmacies would face similar challenges. They would have to maintain a business relationship with 300 different suppliers and process, track, and cut checks to 300 vendors rather than 1 or 2 drug wholesalers. Pharmacies would have to track product use and order needs by supplier. Instead of sending a single order electronically to a single drug wholesaler each evening, the pharmacy would have to deliver separate orders for each supplier. While doable, such activities would take a great deal of staff time and have a real cost to a pharmacy.

If a pharmaceutical manufacturer sells only to drug wholesalers, however, the channel dynamics are quite different. The 60,000-80,000 accounts become no more than 60. The overall number of transactions in the channel using the drug wholesaler model is dramatically lower more than six times lower than would be evident with a direct-channel model.

As an example, consider a drug channel where 70,000 pharmacies order from 300 drug manufacturers. Assume further that these pharmacies order once a week from the 10 largest manufacturers, twice a month from the next 90, monthly from the next 100, and quarterly from the final 100. The total number of orders required to operate the channel on an annual basis using these assumptions is as follows:

70,000 pharmacies $\times$ 52 orders $\times$ 10 manufacturers = 36,400,000 per year

70,000 pharmacies $\times$ 26 orders $\times$ 90 manufacturers = 163,800,000 per year

70,000 pharmacies $\times$ 10 orders $\times$ 100 manufacturers = 70,000,000 per year

70,000 pharmacies $\times$ 4 orders $\times$ 100 manufacturers = 28,000,000 per year

Total channel orders would be 298.2 million transactions. Each purchase transaction also produces four or five additional transactions (e.g., packing slips, invoices, statements, payments, credit and debit memos), so the real transaction total could easily exceed 1.5 billion a year under this model. This result is impressive, despite the fact that the calculations assume a conservative number of customers and ordering cycles. Also consequential is the fact that the direct model would require longer order delivery times and additional inventory investment by pharmacies. And although it would not be a concern for drug manufacturers, a direct-distribution model makes no provision for various auxiliary services.

The drug wholesaler model provides daily delivery to a pharmacy and substantially reduces the number of transactions required to operate the system, thereby reducing costs for both manufacturers and pharmacies and, ultimately, for the American public. Using the same assumptions as before and further assuming that 60 drug wholesalers order on a company basis from drug manufacturers and deliver 255 days a year to pharmacies from 230 distribution centers, total transactions are:

60 wholesalers $\times$ 52 orders $\times$ 10 manufacturers = 31,200
60 wholesalers $\times$ 26 orders $\times$ 90 manufacturers = 140,400
60 wholesalers $\times$ 12 orders $\times$ 100 manufacturers = 72,000
60 wholesalers $\times$ 4 orders $\times$ 100 manufacturers = 24,000

Total drug wholesaler orders to pharmaceutical manufacturers are 267,600. Pharmacy to wholesaler orders would then be:

$$70,000 \text{ pharmacies} \times 255 \text{ orders} \times = 17,850,000$$

The combined total of 18,117,600, or 18.1 million, is only 6% of the total of 298.2 million under the direct model. Looking at it another way, the direct model requires 16.67 times the number of transactions required by the wholesaler model.

From a drug manufacturer's point of view, selling to drug wholesalers rather than directly to all the pharmacies and others is very attractive. The price is generally the same for pharmacy or wholesaler, so the manufacturer gives up no margin. Orders are much larger and therefore more economical to process, pack, and ship. Drug wholesalers are adept at using electronic data interchange, which offers all sorts of efficiencies to both trading partners. Drug wholesalers are physically closer to pharmacies, deliver daily, and provide a whole array of below market cost auxiliary services that pharmacies need to operate effectively.

If a pharmacy runs out of a particular drug manufacturer's product, the drug wholesaler can get it resupplied overnight. Manufacturers shipping direct cannot begin to match this cycle time. For multiple-source products—and increasingly for even sole-source entities—not having the product in stock at the dispensing site means a lost sale for the manufacturer. If this pattern becomes more prevalent, the drug wholesaler model becomes even more important to the drug manufacturer.

## CHALLENGES TO DRUG WHOLESALING

Everyone who takes the time to study today's drug distribution channel comes to the same conclusion: drug wholesalers provide a variety of valuable economic functions and essential commercial services to drug distribution. Further, drug wholesalers operate in such a way that it is actually less expensive and more efficient to use drug wholesalers rather than to order directly from a drug producer or marketer. What also becomes evident to the student of drug wholesaling is that there is no margin left in the business. In fact, drug wholesalers are selling their services (despite the fact that drug products are an integral part of a drug wholesaler's business, drug wholesaling is essentially a service business) at or below commodity price levels. While it is relatively easy to empathize with an industry with little if any margin left, it is more difficult to sustain that empathy when the participants willingly give away what little margin remains by continually ratcheting down their prices.

Current operating margins and returns on investment in mainstream drug wholesaling are not attracting significant capital or new entrants into the marketplace. The reasons are relatively simple: excess capacity coupled with ever-declining margins. The recent spate of consolidations and the first bankruptcies in some time raise the question of whether current operating margins and profitability are sufficient for much of the industry. Whether current operating margins are sustaining margins without further expense reduction is problematic. The issue of sustaining margins is especially pertinent for small to medium companies, but even the largest organizations must address the issue.

Granted, there are efforts under way to design and operate drug distribution centers profitably on 2-3% gross margins, but there are obvious limits to that strategy, too. Tom Peters in *The Pursuit of WOW!* asserts that "If you (or your company) luck out and find something that works, you're in trouble. You'll most likely try to make history repeat itself, which can hardly ever be made to happen." What worked yesterday and even today is rarely what will work tomorrow because circumstances, especially in the drug industry today, continue to change.

Drug wholesalers need a new strategy! The fundamental irony of this statement is what the late W. Edward Demming said in 1993: "The greatest amount of innovation in American business over the next five years will not be in new products, but in distribution and logistics." If correct, drug wholesalers exist in a rich milieu of expectation and opportunity that will help them transform drug wholesaling into its next iteration, a "something new" that commands higher margins and produces sustaining returns.

The second irony is that "something new" will be an even less permanent answer than the low-price, market-share strategy. Transformations are a continuing process; without them an industry will not survive. In *Hypercompetition: Managing the Dynamics of Strategy Maneuvering,* Amos Tuck School of Business professor Richard D'Aveni claims that:

> The new code of conduct is an active strategy of disrupting the status quo to create an unsustainable series of competitive advantages. This is not an age of castles, moats, and armour. It is rather an age of cunning, speed, and surprise. It may be hard for some to hang up the chain mail of sustainable advantage after . . . so many battles. But hypercompetition, a state where sustainable competitive advantages are no longer possible, is now the only level of competition.

A third irony of drug wholesaling is found in its rush to consolidate into fewer, larger companies to take advantage of scale economies and to be in a position to service national health service accounts. While it appears that consolidation helps to reduce overcapacity in drug wholesaling (that continues to worsen with every advance in material handling and distribution logistics technology) and has so far led to profit improvement, consolidation also increases risk for the largest firms. The rush to bigness, according to John Naisbett in *Global Paradox,* creates vulnerability in today's economy. "Big companies and 'economies of scale' succeeded in the comparatively slow-moving decades [leading up to] the mid-1980s. But now, only small and medium-sized companies . . . will survive when we turn the corner of the century." Naisbett predicts further that timely, uncensored information–the kind that large companies are so adept at creating with modern information technology–"will almost certainly put bureaucracies–both in government and commerce–out of business."

For more than four decades, the drug industry was an orderly, predictable industry. Companies competed, but competition bordered on chivalry. No one "got crazy" and few dared to cross traditional boundaries of propriety. Everyone grew accustomed to the notion that the drug industry was an orderly world. In a word, the industry was tidy.

That world is gone–probably forever. What is needed is a little more creative untidiness, which can only occur if enough of the industry gets accustomed to transience as opportunity. As Tom Peter adds, "Tidy times call for tidy strategic schemes. The times aren't tidy, and so our strategic schemes shouldn't be, either."

## A FINAL NOTE

Drug wholesalers are clearly the best at what they do, and they do a lot for the drug industry and the American public. It is also obvious that the marketplace, both manufacturers and the drug wholesalers' customers, is getting a great deal for very little. What is becoming more evident is that drug wholesalers need to find new avenues for competitive advantage, that new advantages will be transient, and that it is possible that being very large may not be the advantage some believe it to be. Drug wholesalers have shown a remarkable resilience and ability to change throughout their long history. Time will tell if these traits still lurk in the industry's gene pool.

# Prospects for Pharmaceutical Promotion

## William G. Castagnoli

*Those who cannot remember the past are condemned to repeat it.*
                                                    – George Santayana

### INTRODUCTION

This often quoted aphorism warning of adverse consequences for those who neglect to study the past would appear inappropriate in a discussion of pharmaceutical promotion prospects, for nothing in the history of pharmaceutical advertising and promotion in the United States had prepared the industry, its advertising agencies, and the suppliers of communication services for the abrupt promotion decline that occurred in 1993 and 1994.

From the mid-1950s, when the pharmaceutical renaissance began, until 1993, manufacturers' expenditures in advertising, promotion, and communication programs had grown steadily. Field forces had gone from hundreds to thousands of representatives and journal ads from single-page displays of product packaging to colorful multipage units. Hundreds of new publications were launched to satisfy the demand for space. An array of new promotional vehicles was created: advertising on prescription pads and health record forms; audio- and videotapes for car, office, and home; cable TV; FM radio; instructional programs in a variety of formats, etc. All of these were aimed at registering the industry's messages with prescribers. The remarkable growth in U.S. pharmaceutical sales from $1.3 billion

William G. Castagnoli is Contributing Editor, *Medical Marketing & Media*, 126 Soundview Terrace, Northport, NY 11768.

[Haworth co-indexing entry note]: "Prospects for Pharmaceutical Promotion." Castagnoli, William G. Co-published simultaneously in *Journal of Pharmaceutical Marketing & Management* (Pharmaceutical Products Press, an imprint of The Haworth Press, Inc.) Vol. 10, No. 4, 1996, pp. 223-235; and: *Pharmaceutical Marketing in the 21st Century* (ed: Mickey C. Smith) Pharmaceutical Products Press, an imprint of The Haworth Press, Inc., 1996, pp. 223-235. Single or multiple copies of this article are available from The Haworth Document Delivery Service [1-800-342-9678, 9:00 a.m. - 5:00 p.m. (EST)].

*223*

in 1954 to $54.8 billion in 1994 supported the burgeoning growth in advertising and promotion (1, 2).

Then, in 1993, the virtually straight-line trend of some 40 years encountered new, threatening circumstances well-known to observers of the pharmaceutical industry. The unrelenting rise in health care costs became a pressing concern for individuals and businesses, and this concern translated into a political movement to restructure the health delivery system. In the debate over health care, the prices of pharmaceuticals were pushed center stage as a major part of the problem. New providers – managed care organizations (MCOs) and pharmaceutical benefit managers (PBMs) – emerged as cost-saving answers. Most important, the pharmaceutical industry, suddenly under unprecedented pressure to hold down prices and envisioning a dramatically changing sales environment, pulled back on promotion. With a questionable future and many companies influenced by unpromising research pipelines, the industry chose to retrench promotionally. Advertising and promotional expenditures, along with all budgetary items, came under scrutiny and, with everything else, were reduced.

As this is being written in early 1995, national health care reform has been defeated. A probusiness attitude is resident in Congress, and managing health has been tossed to the states. Considerable concern over rising health care costs remains, and managed care has been accepted as the answer to holding down health care cost escalation. Accordingly, the MCO market is the new, pressing reality. Pharmaceutical companies are endeavoring to adjust to a new way of doing business. The question: Was the 1993 downturn a blip or the beginning of a fundamental change in advertising and promotional programs by the industry? Before attempting to answer this question, it is advisable, given Santayana's admonition, to consider the elements that encouraged a robust promotional environment in the past.

## FACTORS FAVORING PROMOTION

### Communication Obligations on Pharmaceuticals

If a drug is to be used properly, it must be accompanied by an envelope of information. The truism that a pill, capsule, or vial is worthless, or even dangerous, without identification and instruction is worth repeating, for it emphasizes the responsibility manufacturers have to prescribers and patients. It follows, then, that there is a marketing mandate for thorough communication. Witness the industry's basic promotional/communication technique: the face-to-face meeting of prescriber and company representative. What could be more ideal for an information exchange?

In short, a crucial aspect of pharmaceutical marketing is that it goes beyond selling the competitive advantages of the product to the need for an information transfer. Accordingly, the "promotional" budget covers such activities as seminars, conferences, product monographs, and instructional information on diagnosis and treatment. These are only promotional in the sense that they are product connected. These items contribute significantly to the expense of marketing a pharmaceutical.

## Competitive Intensity

High levels of promotion are a sign of a competitive marketplace, not characteristic of monopolies or oligopolies. Considering that there are over 30 major players in the U.S. market, with no single company approaching a 10% share, the promotional intensity of the past 40 years follows logically. Even given the acquisitions and mergers that have occurred during this period, the creation of new biotech companies and the arrival of sizeable overseas manufacturers (Glaxo, Hoechst, and Bayer, for example) have maintained the competitive pitch of the market.

## Brand Obsolescence

Central to promotional activity in pharmaceuticals is the technological nature of the industry. New products emerge continually from research to displace or challenge existing brands. In this churning environment, return on investment must be gained as quickly as possible before the product encounters its equivalent or its successor. This process encourages heavy promotional emphasis on introduction to break through existing prescribing habits and, once established, to maximize sales.

Adding to this need to infuse promotional stimulus into the brand's life cycle is the looming date of genericization. Once the product is off patent, promotion is cut drastically. Genericization is a significant influence in reducing promotion once the product has become a commodity, but it also encourages high levels of activity as the manufacturer endeavors to maximize return during the years that the product is single source.

## Value of Individual Prescribers

It is doubtful whether any other industry has sold its products to the breadth of significant individual customers as the U.S. pharmaceutical industry has in the past 40 years in the U.S. High-volume practices generated hundreds of thousands of dollars in sales in widely applicable drug categories–antibiotics, psychotropics, antiarthritics, and antihypertensives, for example. This meant that considerable funds could be spent on individual prescribers in the form of repeated sales calls, educational/instructional materials, patient aids and service items, and a myriad of reminder devices.

The typical prescribing base on a brand (primary care M.D.s plus specialty groups) usually totalled 75,000-100,000 individuals. This number provided an audience of unique size, one small enough for individual attention by a sales force of 1,000 representatives but still broad enough to allow for the efficiencies of mass media (medical journals, direct mail, public relations, cable TV, etc.). This audience dimension was congenial to proliferation of communication and promotional devices–everything from closed-circuit TV conferences to logo coffee cups–as pharmaceutical company competition added to the depth of the promotional stream.

These were the major influences behind the promotional acceleration that the industry has experienced since the mid-1950s. In the pivotal year 1993, the trend reversed as the nation became concerned with the cost of health care and focused its attention on pharmaceuticals. It will be useful to review some statistics reflecting what happened to promotional activity recently before considering prospects for the future, once again following the advice about remembering the past.

## SPENDING PATTERNS IN THE 1990s

### Field Force Size

The number of sales representatives employed by pharmaceutical companies grew steadily in the decades prior to 1990. For managerial reasons and sales focus, some companies, in expanding, organized their field forces into separate units. Examples are Glaxo (Allen & Hanburys, Cerenex, Glaxo Pharmaceutical, Glaxo Dermatology), Pfizer (Pfizer Labs, Roerig, Pratt), Merck (Groups I, II, III). Many operated specialized forces for such areas as pediatrics, oncology, and psychiatry. In 1992, the 32 biggest prescription firms had reached the aggregate total of 42,771 sales representatives (3).

Appreciation of the need to reduce sales force size had surfaced prior to 1993, but the reductions that did occur at some companies were offset by increases at others, so even with an anticipation of a storm ahead, there was a 12% increase in the total between 1990 and 1992. In 1992, the need to downsize hit home so that by the end of 1994 the total had fallen to 36,792–a 12% decrease.

Notable reductions were Bristol-Myers Squibb (–30%), Berlex (–6%), CIBA (–36%), Hoechst (–24%), Lederle (–55%), Parke-Davis (–30%), Sandoz (–25%), Searle (–7%), SmithKline Beecham (–12%), Syntex (–69%), Upjohn (–34%), Zeneca (–24%), Knoll (–12%), Eli Lilly (–5%), and Johnson & Johnson (–5%). The result in this reduction in field forces is seen in an IMS report on sales calls (Table 1).

While the number of traditional sales force representatives has declined, the numbers of representatives assigned to managed care organizations has increased. From 1990 to 1992, this total advanced 26%. In 1993, the increase among the 22 most active companies was over 100%! In 1994, that spectacular pace had cooled to a less startling 22%.

These MCO percentages, of course, are on small bases and also include additions to the regional account managers' rosters. This restructuring of sales departments is aimed at MCOs so that categorization does reflect emphasis on these new customers. For perspective, the largest managed care forces are Merck (80), Glaxo (80), Marion Merrell Dow (60), Abbott (60), Johnson & Johnson (57), and SmithKline Beecham (43).

Additionally, another MCO-oriented sales group are representatives assigned to HMOs and PPOs. Called "pull-through reps," these representatives are charged with encouraging adherence to drug formularies among staff model physicians. Some totals are available: Pfizer (29), SmithKline Beecham (21), and Lilly (17).

## *Medical Journal Advertising*

Journals serving the managed care market have attracted more advertising recently, and some new ones directed at MCO audiences have been launched, but minor positives here have not come near making up for the major negatives in advertising revenue reported by medical journals. Probably influenced more by cost-cutting decisions than judgments that broadscale advertising to physicians was no longer effective, pharmaceuti-

| TABLE 1. Sales Calls in Millions (4). | | | |
|---|---|---|---|
| Year | Office | Service | Hospital |
| 1993 | 24.5 | 10.3 | 8.0 |
| 1994 | 21.7 | 9.5 | 7.1 |
| % Change | –11% | –7% | –11% |

cal advertisers pulled back on journal space in 1993. Consider HCI's audit of advertising expenditures (Table 2). In the first half of 1994, many of the leading publications in the field experienced sizeable dips in income (6):

| | |
|---|---|
| *Medical Economics* | –21.5% |
| *Journal of the American Medical Association* | –24.8% |
| *New England Journal of Medicine* | –27.5% |
| *Postgraduate Medicine* | –22.3% |

### Direct-to-Consumer Advertising (DTC)

While detailing and journal advertising have, of late, experienced re-ductions in spending, a relative newcomer to pharmaceutical promotion, direct-to-consumer advertising through print, radio, and TV, has been growing. The technique was initiated in the early 1980s and has come into its own in the mid-1990s.

A good deal of this advertising has been disease-oriented–nonbranded messages directing consumers to see their doctor about a medical condition. This approach has been widely used on television, where regulatory restric-tions make brand-name promotion in conjunction with a disease indication prohibitively expensive by requiring the inclusion of disclosure text in the message. The format of newspapers and magazines, however, allows enough space to carry disclosure information economically and, accordingly, there has been an explosion of DTC advertising in these media.

It must be pointed out that DTC, although used by a range of compa-

| TABLE 2. Advertising Expenditures in Health Care Journals (5). | | |
|---|---|---|
| Year | $(000) | % Change |
| 1991 | 482,976 | +12.0 |
| 1992 | 641,534 | +32.8 |
| 1993 | 571,564 | –10.9 |
| 1994 | 556,564 | –2.7 |

nies, displays, from time to time, a concentration of ads on a certain disease category. For example, the companies marketing nicotine patches invested heavily in name registration and reminder advertising on TV and in print in 1992. Currently, Abbot's Hytrin® and Merck's Proscar® are in a well-funded head-to-head competition for benign prostatic hypertrophy (BPH) using both nonbranded disease-oriented messages and branded messages. Together the two companies are greatly heightening the public's awareness of prostate disease while pursuing their own commercial interests. The trend in DTC is shown in audited reports on advertising spending from Leading National Advertisers (Table 3).

It can be pointed out that the increase in DTC compensates in part for the reduction in medical journal advertising in the totality of industry promotional spending. Furthermore, the audited data do not report on follow-up activities such as direct mail, events, and consumer discounts, which round out DTC programs in replying to inquiries to TV or print offers. Upjohn's Rogaine® program is illustrative of how extensive the "relationship marketing" phase of DTC can be, with consumers receiving not only a packet of brochures and sales literature on Rogaine but also a list of dermatologists available (at reduced cost to the patient) for a consultation on the product and hair loss.

## *Meetings and Events*

Estimates of the content and expenditures of pharmaceutical companies in meetings and events have not been informed by audits comparable to the detailing and journal services. Companies specializing in scientific and educational programs for health care audiences have made educated guesses over the years as to the dimensions of company investment in such

| TABLE 3. Expenditures in DTC Advertising ($ Millions) (7). | | | |
|---|---|---|---|
| Year | Corporate and Nonbranded | Branded | Total |
| 1990 | N/A | 47.0 | 47.0 |
| 1991 | 9.7 | 55.8 | 65.5 |
| 1992 | 33.2 | 156.2 | 189.4 |
| 1993 | 52.6 | 130.4 | 183.0 |
| 1994* | 63.3 | 187.4 | 250.7 |

* January-September only

activities as symposia, dinner meetings, continuing medical education (CME) courses, telephone and video conferences and the outreach materials (transcripts, literature reviews, reprints, patient aids, etc.) generated by these activities, but no hard numbers have been available.

Scott-Levin Associates launched Physicians Meeting and Events Audit (PMEA) last year reporting on 1993 by surveying a sample of physicians projectable to an audience of 69,000. PMEA estimated $494,450 had been spent in 1993. The survey just completed for 1994 and projecting to an audience of 79,000 shows a 25% increase to $543,750 (8).

These meetings would place expenditures on meetings and events markedly counter to detailing and journal advertising. Without audits for the early 1990s, however, we do not know whether the 1993 and 1994 levels represent reductions from previous highs.[1] A 25% increase would certainly indicate anything but a contraction in the use of this phase of marketing. However, there is a factor clouding the picture on meetings and events.

In 1991, the FDA proposed rules for continuing medical education that would greatly complicate the managing of such activities by commercial sponsors. The proposed guidelines, which have yet to be formalized, together with pronouncements by FDA officials on the need to curb product promotion in CME and enforcement action by FDA on the distribution by companies of educational materials that contained reference to products and unapproved indications, produced the proverbial "chilling effect" on CME-related meetings and events. Anecdotal reports indicate that a spending freeze pending resolution of what was and was not allowed occurred in the industry. So it is that we do not know whether 1993 at $494,450 was a reduction from previous years or a recovery from a previous low in 1992 influenced by the FDA enforcement policy. The FDA action occurred just when economy moves and cautious attitudes could easily have justified a shifting of funds from meeting and events to other media, even journals, which in 1992 showed a sizeable increase. Also, we can question whether 1994 at $543,750 is an advance over the early 1990s or simply a return to the norm of that period.

Regardless of these doubts as to trends, with a 25% increase in 1994, meetings and events appear to be in favor currently in the promotional/communications mix for pharmaceuticals.

### Other Health Care Audience Media

A comprehensive picture of the recent history of pharmaceutical promotion would be incomplete without a review of the considerable number of techniques used by pharmaceutical marketers in addition to detailing, journal ads, DTC, and meetings/events. If the latter has presented a statistical void, this catchall category is an informational black hole. To fill the gap, HCI has just initiated a "nonjournal" report, beginning with a survey of 1994. HCI's figure for that year is $125,032,000.[2]

Without a reference point from previous years, it is impossible to assess what this figure represents as to trends, but it is hard to imagine companies in a cost-cutting phase reducing journal and field force expenditures and not also dropping budgets in this category. There were some outstanding reductions as well. Medical News Network (MNN), the Whittle TV news service for physicians, ballooned the financial expenditure in this group with investments from sponsors in 1992-1993 of more than $100,000,000. MNN closed its doors in 1994 when it was unable to obtain sufficient financial commitments to expand beyond a demonstration project with 5,000 physicians. Similarly, Lifetime Medical Television's Sunday programming for physicians went off the air, displaced by more profitable consumer fare. American Medical Television, the AMA competition to Lifetime, has also been discontinued. All of these TV programs represented sizeable budgetary allocations from pharmaceutical advertisers in time and production costs. They have all gone dark, not from a lack of viewership but from industry belt-tightening and reallocation of resources.

The demise of MD television enterprises, which had relied on advertising revenues from the pharmaceutical industry, has not discouraged attempts to use the most pervasive communication medium of our society to reach physicians. As this is being written, Physician Television Network is planning to begin broadcasting in July 1995 using the new Hughes satellite, which will beam programs to subscribers with an 18-inch receiver dish. Television figures prominently in planning health-oriented media for consumers. American Health Network is only one of a dozen or more advertiser-supported endeavors now on the drawing boards for launch in 1995 on cable TV. Likely advertisers are pharmaceutical companies with DTC campaigns.

The boundless potential of the computer has attracted entrepreneurs, academe, medical organizations, hospitals, and advertisers interested in its capacity for information retrieval, communication, interactive interchange, and promotion. Numerous local experiments by medical schools, hospitals, MCOs, and physician groups are under way.

Examples of advertiser-supported computer services are GeoMedica, scheduled for testing in 1995, and Physicians OnLine, a going concern with 40,000 users and Marion Merrell Dow, Astra/Merck, and Sandoz as sponsors (9).

## PROSPECTS FOR PHARMACEUTICAL PROMOTION

Having "remembered" the past (factors encouraging strenuous pharmaceutical promotion) and recent events (promotional spending patterns in the 1990s), the question remains: Will we "repeat" pre-1993 history as so many in the promotional industry would be willing to be "condemned" to do, or is the promotional side of the business due for significant change?

Students of evolution have argued whether species change gradually or suddenly. Some find in the fossil record evidence that major changes in skeletal structure, breathing, and feeling organs, for example, came about rapidly in response to sudden catastrophic events that so altered the environment that life had to change radically to survive. Accepting the premise that radical change comes from radical cause and applying this principle to our question about the direction of pharmaceutical promotion, we must ask: Has the pharmaceutical selling environment changed so drastically as to force the promotional function to be transformed? My feeling is that it has not.

I still see on the scene the pressing need for in-depth communication between company and prescriber. What about formulary instructions and treatment guidelines in managed care organizations? Will not information necessary to the proper use of drugs be provided by noncommercial sources? It doesn't seem to be working out that way. MCOs are using company salespeople who represent drugs on formulary to inform and promote on the MCOs' formularies because the company representatives know the products thoroughly and are motivated to stimulate prescribing; these are the pull-through representatives cited earlier. Moreover, MCOs are even employing promotional campaigns to educate and remind physicians within their organizations to stay within the MCOs' formularies (10). This commercial approach is required because physician prerogatives must be maintained for good M.D. morale and cooperation and for acceptable medical practice. Because one or two drugs do not fit all patients, a formulary must have breadth. With breadth comes choice, and choice is the basis of promotion. In short, someone has to discharge the communication mandate, and I see a continuing role for pharmaceutical companies to do it.

Earlier, I advanced the premise that intense competition fosters promotional intensity. I see no reason to believe that competition will be markedly less in the future than it is today. Consolidation will reduce the number of corporate entities, but even if we doubled up all the major companies in the U.S. by the year 2000, we would still have more than a dozen sizeable competitors contending for market share.

I also believe that the technological nature of pharmaceuticals lowers the barriers to entry into the business. It is still possible for a small laboratory to hit upon a crucial scientific discovery, license or produce a product, and without heavy capital investment or distribution clout, add itself to the competitive mosaic of the industry. There are certainly enough bright minds and investors out there to do just that. Ergo: continuing competition from the bottom up.

As for the push that brand obsolescence gives to promotion, the situation is unchanged. If anything, company consolidations create larger corporations which will have the resources and the need to exploit a product to the fullest throughout the patent-protected period of its life cycle.

If three factors encouraging promotion in the past–information need, competition, and drug obsolescence–are essentially the same, the fourth–prescribing audience–has undergone significant change. The decision-making/prescribing entity has contracted and undergone a mind shift. The new players are the MCO and PBM formulary managers who have drawn off power from physicians. Tens of thousands of M.D.s are still writing scripts, but their selections of drugs are coming under the purview of a few thousand managers interested in cost and not therapeutic preference. It has been this audience definition (along with the prospects of lower profits from lower prices to MCOs) that has led to field force reductions and cuts in journal space. The industry's reflexive reaction as been, Why do across-the-board promotion if MCO bidding is the new marketing model?

I do not believe that the audience reconfiguration the industry is now experiencing will spell the end of traditional promotional methods or the long-term positive trend in promotion. It will take a few years for the marketing departments to learn how to deal with this new buying procedure, but the adjustment will be made. Companies are already experienced in selling to hospitals and buying groups under formulary systems and have been effective in this venue. Also, as previously noted, the pull-through process of drugs on formulary is beginning to be recognized, and I see this activity as growing in importance as a promotional technique. Selling to managed care (with its restrictions on sales reps' activities, literature distribution, etc.) is certainly a more restrictive promotional environment, but for me, this represents a restriction in degree and not a change in the methods employed.

Keeping traditional promotion alive will be the continuation of private practice. As evidenced by European socialized medicine, a managed system may dominate, but there remains a place for private practice. America's impatience with regimentation, its wealth, and the varied pattern of health care delivery that is evolving all bode well for private practice surviving and representing a significant share of the pharmaceutical market.

The downturn in promotion experienced in 1993 and 1994 was caused, in part, by the threat of price controls implicit in federal health care "reform." That specter has departed. Additionally, the expanding regulatory actions of an activist FDA were a depressing influence on promotion, particularly on meetings and events. As with health care reform, a political change has reduced this negative, and in fact, with a movement afoot to restructure the FDA to make it less hostile to industry, the climate for promotion may be improved.

## CONCLUSIONS

All things considered, the prospects for promotion can be described as cautiously optimistic. Optimism is based on the belief that the influences for healthy promotion–informational need, intense competition, and product obsolescence–remain. The one major change–audience redefinition–should not derail the industry's promotional impulse, only reroute it.

Growth in DTC (spending at a $330 million rate in 1994) is more than making up for the downturn in medical journal advertising. And with DTC come follow-up programs to consumers, which although not audited, undoubtedly add considerably to this spending category. Meetings and events, based on the 25% increase in 1994, are reviving as industry learns to live with the FDA's "preliminary" CME guidelines. This essential informational activity in pharmaceutical communications should grow further if legal efforts (the Washington Legal Foundation's suit) to reverse the FDA's CME policy are successful.

Overall optimism on promotion envisions the maintenance of good-sized sales forces to service managed care (formulary sales and pull-through detailing) and a private practice market, respectable levels of journal advertising as a promotional backdrop, increasing budgets for meetings and events, growing investment in DTC and related consumer programs, and experimental support for new media.

The perfunctory cautious note is added as homage to Santayana's advice. The size of the 1993-1994 downturn was not presaged by previous events. It represented the unexpected. History teaches respect for the unexpected.

## NOTES

1. In an analysis of pharmaceutical promotion prepared by the American Association of Advertising Agencies (AAAA), "Medical Informational Services (symposia, meetings, publication and conventions)" had been approximated at $700 million for 1992.

2. HCI's *Medical Promotion Audit (MPA), 1995 Non-Journal Report* includes television for physicians, "desk top" media, and waiting room media.

## REFERENCES

1. U.S. Department of Commerce.

2. Pharmaceutical Research and Manufacturers Association (PhRMA).

3. Scott-Levin Associates. Sales force structure & strategies 1994. Statistics on sales force sizes and their decreases and increases are from this text.

4. IMS. Year-in-review, 1995.

5. HCI. Medical Promotion Audit (MPA), 1995.

6. Advertising Age 1994;(Aug 29).

7. Leading National Advertisers. Media watch multi-media service, 1994.

8. Scott-Levin Associates. Physician Meeting and Event Audit (PMEA), 1994.

9. Holliday L. New media report card: where are we now? Med Market Media 1995;30(Feb):46-56.

10. Castagnoli WG. Hold it! Don't kill the sales budget. Med Market Media 1994;29(Apr):12-8.

# The Impact of Current Trends in Health Care on the Pharmaceutical Sales Force of the Future

James E. Dutton
Michelle A. Reece

## INTRODUCTION

The rapidly occurring changes in the health care environment of the last few years have had a profound impact on the pharmaceutical industry and the role of its sales representatives. After years of rapid growth and expansion, multiple factors are now influencing the way in which pharmaceutical companies compete in today's marketplace. The primary catalysts for change have been the growing prevalence of managed health care and the push toward health care reform. These, in turn, have increased the focus on pricing issues and the importance of showing the value of drug products through pharmacoeconomics and outcomes research. This emphasis on cost-effectiveness is expected to increase as health care in this country evolves toward various forms of managed care such as HMOs, PPOs, MCOs, IPAs, totally integrated health care systems, and disease management systems.

James E. Dutton, M.S., C.M.R., is President of Certified Medical Representatives Institute, Inc., 4950 Brambleton Avenue, Roanoke, VA 24018. Michelle A. Reece, M.Ed., is Curriculum Coordinator at Certified Medical Representatives Institute, Inc.

[Haworth co-indexing entry note]: "The Impact of Current Trends in Health Care on the Pharmaceutical Sales Force of the Future." Dutton, James E., and Michelle A. Reece. Co-published simultaneously in *Journal of Pharmaceutical Marketing & Management* (Pharmaceutical Products Press, an imprint of The Haworth Press, Inc.) Vol. 10, No. 4, 1996, pp. 237-250; and: *Pharmaceutical Marketing in the 21st Century* (ed: Mickey C. Smith) Pharmaceutical Products Press, an imprint of The Haworth Press, Inc., 1996, pp. 237-250. Single or multiple copies of this article are available from The Haworth Document Delivery Service [1-800-342-9678, 9:00 a.m. - 5:00 p.m. (EST)].

## BACKGROUND

The traditional role of pharmaceutical sales representatives has undergone tremendous change as a result of this evolution within the health care industry. As recently as the 1980s, health care in this country existed primarily as a fee-for-service industry. Historically, the primary target audience for pharmaceutical sales representatives wishing to market their drug products was the fee-for-service physician (1). Selling strategies were product oriented and highlighted the benefits of their products over those of the closest competitors. Compensation packages for representatives were based almost exclusively on the volume of products sold in a given sales territory. In most areas of the country today, however, these practices are becoming the exception rather than the rule. The two most prominent trends of the early 1990s, the growth of managed health care and health care reform, have resulted in many of the significant changes being seen in the pharmaceutical industry today.

## INFLUENCE OF MANAGED CARE AND HEALTH CARE REFORM

The phenomenal growth in managed care organizations has been occurring since the mid-1980s, initially as a response to the need to contain escalating health care costs in this country. More recently, however, this rapid growth has been fueled by several key factors, including federal and state government initiatives, the anticipation of national health care reform, and private sector initiatives such as the increasing entry of insurance companies and large employers into the managed care market. As late as 1984, managed health care plans accounted for only 11% of the health-insured population. By 1987, approximately 56% of this same population was enrolled in a type of managed care plan. Since then, these numbers have continued to grow, and by 1997, less than 10% of the health-insured population is expected to be covered by traditional fee-for-service plans (2).

The success of managed health care during recent years is reflected in both the growing number of enrollees nationwide and the increasing competition between managed care organizations. Although the total number of managed care organizations has declined recently due to consolidation within the industry, the number of enrollees within these organizations has continued to grow. Between 1986 and 1993, the number of enrollees in health maintenance organizations (HMOs) grew from 26 million to nearly

49 million. The number of enrollees covered by preferred provider organizations (PPOs) also has continued to grow, approaching 60 million covered lives in 1993 (3, 4). Strong market penetration has continued in most areas of the country, with the exception of the South Central region (Texas, Oklahoma, Arkansas, Louisiana, Mississippi, Alabama, Tennessee, and Kentucky). States that currently have the highest market penetration include Massachusetts (38.9%), California (36.4%), Maryland (34.5%), Minnesota (33.6%), Oregon (30.4%), and Colorado (28.7%) (5). The tremendous impact of this growth in managed care on pharmaceutical sales representatives will be discussed further in a later section.

The second primary trend of the 1990s influencing health care in this country was the introduction of proposed legislation for health care reform by the Clinton Administration. This resulted in an intense focus on health care issues and led to the creation and introduction of numerous other reform proposals. Although legislation in any form has yet to materialize, the impact of this discourse on the pharmaceutical industry was profound. Health care reform became the impetus for many of the same changes in the pharmaceutical industry that had already occurred in other industries during the 1980s (e.g., corporate downsizing of the industry as a whole and concurrent shrinking sales forces).

As the pricing policies of the pharmaceutical industry came under attack by Congress and the Clinton Administration, the importance of showing the value of the industry's pharmaceutical products intensified. This has been accomplished most successfully through the new emphasis on pharmacoeconomic studies, outcomes research, and quality-of-life studies, which show the benefits of pharmaceuticals over more costly, invasive procedures and the cost-effectiveness of one drug over another. This shift in focus to the economic aspects of pharmaceuticals has resulted in considerable changes in the training and education required for today's pharmaceutical sales reps. It has also resulted in several important trends prevalent today within the industry.

## RECENT DEVELOPMENTS IN THE INDUSTRY

The pharmaceutical industry as a whole has been undergoing change at a rapid pace over the last two years, and it continues to evolve. Several recent developments are likely to shape the industry well into the future. These developments include the recent and continuing mergers of individual pharmaceutical companies, the acquisition of or strategic alliances with pharmacy benefit management companies (PBMs) by pharmaceutical companies, the partial shift of research and development from pharmaceutical companies to biotechnology firms, the development of integrated health care delivery systems, and the new emphasis on disease management. Some companies also are creating regional business units that will allow them to have greater flexibility and to move faster in making changes and responding to the changing marketplace.

Recent acquisitions among pharmaceutical companies, with more currently in negotiation, are resulting in fewer but larger companies. Since November of 1993, 9 major pharmaceutical corporations have purchased other pharmaceutical companies or pharmacy benefit management companies. These recent acquisitions are listed in Table 1.

The acquisitions of pharmaceutical companies by other pharmaceutical companies include Syntex by Roche, Sterling Winthrop (OTC products only) by SmithKline and Bayer, and American Cyanamid by American Home Products. The acquisition of Chiron (a biotechnology company) by CIBA-GEIGY, a pharmaceutical company, represents a trend that is likely to continue in the future. The acquisitions of PBMs by pharmaceutical companies include Medco Containment Services by Merck & Co., Diversified Pharmaceutical Services by SmithKline Beecham, and PCS Health Systems by Eli Lilly. In addition, Pfizer recently formed a strategic alliance with Value Health. Currently being negotiated are the acquisition of Wellcome by Glaxo and Marion Merrell Dow by Hoechst. The creation of these new industry giants will likely produce further cost-cutting measures within the industry.

Some industry experts predict that these recent mergers may affect drug companies' research and development efforts in a negative way. Factors in

TABLE 1

| Drug Industry Acquisitions | | |
|---|---|---|
| Date | Acquiring Company | Target Company |
| November 1993 | Merck & Co. | Medco Containment Services |
| May 1994 | Smith Kline Beecham | Diversified Pharmaceutical Services |
| August 1994 | Sandoz | Gerber Products |
| October 1994 | Roche Holding | Syntex |
| November 1994 | Smith Kline and Bayer | Sterling Winthrop (OTC products) |
| November 1994 | American Home Products | American Cyanamid |
| November 1994 | Eli Lilly | PCS Health Systems |
| January 1995 | CIBA–GEIGY | Chiron |
| Proposed | Glaxo | Wellcome |
| In Negotiations | Hoechst | Marion Merrell Dow |

the current health care environment are changing the traditional approach to pharmaceutical research, development, and marketing. This is causing some pharmaceutical companies to adapt their strategies to accommodate the changing environment. One possible scenario is that these large pharmaceutical companies may eventually rely on small biotechnology firms for the majority of their breakthrough research, with the potential breakthrough drug being marketed under licensing arrangements (6). Perhaps most important, these recent acquisitions and mergers also have helped provide the means for pharmaceutical companies to move into the area of disease management.

Disease management has become a major new area of focus and opportunity for the pharmaceutical industry. Total disease management is an approach to patient care that focuses on the overall course of the disease, as opposed to the traditional approach, which focuses on individual therapeutic interventions. To ensure the delivery of the highest quality of care in the most cost-effective manner, total disease management incorporates tools, such as clinical practice guidelines, to improve patient outcomes (7). By focusing patient management on the optimal treatment strategy, disease management attempts to improve upon the traditional strategies of managing health care processes and costs.

Pharmaceutical companies have a unique opportunity to position themselves as key players in the movement toward disease management systems. To some extent, companies are moving away from reliance on the development of new breakthrough drugs to the development of a package of services for health care providers that includes prevention, diagnosis, treatment, and value-added services and programs (7). This emphasis on providing a comprehensive package of services is resulting in the formation of long-term relationships with key health care providers; these relationships focus on increasing the efficacy of patient care. The new emphasis is also causing the marketing strategies of companies to become more focused on the clinical, economic, and humanistic value of drugs and how these products can be used to treat a disease over its entire course. The introduction of disease management systems may also cause companies to form alliances with PBMs or to purchase PBMs to increase their market share within these systems. Many pharmaceutical companies today are being required to offer volume discounts to health care organizations or to share financial risk in capitated systems where there are contracts based on usage. This will have a significant impact on pharmaceutical representatives, as they will need to acquire a considerably broader knowledge base and to learn to work with new decision makers.

Another recent development in the industry represents a major shift in the way in which health care is delivered in the United States. The development of integrated health care systems goes beyond traditional managed care systems and is considered by many to be, in effect, the second revolution in health care delivery, with the proliferation of managed health care being the first. The term integrated health care system, or IHS, refers to the banding together of health care providers (physicians, hospitals, HMOs, nursing homes, etc.) as a means of coordinating patient care, strengthening or broadening the range of services offered, expanding geographic coverage, and more successfully competing for managed care contracts (5). The goal of these alliances is to create a "seamless continuum" of health services, integrating all aspects of care–primary through tertiary–into a medically and financially accountable health care system.

Provider integration has evolved in direct response to managed care, closely trailing the growth and geographic distribution of managed care activity nationwide. Integrated health care systems are today being developed or considered in nearly every major metropolitan area and in many smaller cities across the U.S. According to one recent survey, nearly 57% of hospitals, 77% of multihospital systems, and 45% of physician group practices have created integrated systems or plan to do so in the near future (5). Regardless of the degree of provider integration, all integrated systems are designed around the basic imperative of accepting substantial medical and financial responsibility for the population they serve. For most IHSs, this implies a number of key elements, including comprehensive medical services, orientation to total disease management, broad geographic coverage, shared risks, shared incentives, physician leadership, advanced information systems to coordinate patient care, capitation-based contracts, total quality management, and a common ownership/management structure. The five most common IHS organizational models include the group practice without walls (GPWW), the physician-hospital organization (PHO), the management services organization model (MSO), the medical foundation model, and the fully integrated provider network (5). Pharmaceutical representatives working within these integrated systems will need a strong knowledge base and a thorough understanding of how their IHSs operate. They will also need to develop with their companies specific and unique strategies for selling their products within these systems.

## CURRENT SALES FORCE SIZE TRENDS

The pharmaceutical industry sales force has undergone significant changes in both the total number of representatives in the field and the necessary skills required for reps to excel in their position. Most companies have downsized their sales forces to some extent since the latter half of 1991, and this trend has continued to the present. This came subsequent to a significant expansion in the size of the average sales force during the mid- to late 1980s, with all of the largest pharmaceutical companies either increasing or maintaining the size of their sales force during this period (8). The reduction in pharmaceutical sales force numbers has continued into 1995. According to a study by Scott-Levin Associates Inc., the industry's top 32 companies reduced their sales force by 700 representatives during the early part of 1995 (9). The trend in the size of the sales force (including managed care and government affairs reps), is illustrated in Figure 1. There has also been a downward trend in the number of reps calling exclusively on physicians. This trend is illustrated in Figure 2.

While it is yet uncertain whether the ranks of pharmaceutical reps will continue to decline or remain steady, it is highly unlikely that the total numbers will ever increase again to the peak levels of 1992. However, it is certain that pharmaceutical representatives will continue to play an integral role in the selling and marketing of pharmaceuticals over the next 10 to 15 years.

## *IMPLICATIONS OF CURRENT TRENDS FOR PHARMACEUTICAL REPS*

Today's pharmaceutical sales rep requires an increased knowledge and skill base to compete successfully in the rapidly changing health care

FIGURE 1

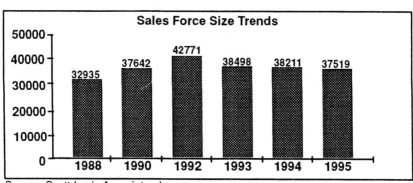

Source: Scott-Levin Associates Inc.

FIGURE 2

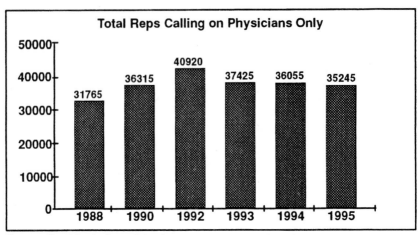

Source: Scott-Levin Associates Inc.

environment. Multiple factors such as the prevalence of managed health care systems, the growth of integrated health care systems, the increased emphasis on pharmacoeconomics, and the emergence of total disease management systems are influencing the role of pharmaceutical sales representatives.

The rapid proliferation of managed health care and integrated health care systems has greatly diminished the relative influence of the physician as the primary sales target (10). This trend can be expected to continue, and the resources and manpower devoted strictly to providing sales calls for traditional fee-for-service physicians will likely decline simultaneously (5). This is due in large part to industry trends, which show that the leading pharmaceutical manufacturers derive roughly half of their U.S. drug revenues from bulk purchases by large provider networks, and many industry analysts expect this percentage to increase in the years ahead (5). For the pharmaceutical representative, integrated health care systems will present new challenges within a sometimes unfamiliar environment. Disease management also creates new challenges for companies compensating reps who are selling in an environment where increased volume sales may not always benefit the company.

These trends have created a need for sales reps who are qualified to sell to a constantly changing target audience. Today's sales person increasingly will be asked to call on managed care organizations within a territory and to work with national accounts representatives as well as call on individual physicians and pharmacists (11). As a result, education and training requirements have also changed. Today's pharmaceutical industry sales executives are more likely to be looking for candidates with a business degree rather than degrees in biology or science (12). This trend is likely to continue as business skills become increasingly important in the current selling environment.

The shift away from traditional person-to-person sales efforts to business-to-system negotiations will result in resources being directed into high-level negotiations with key IHS and managed care decision makers. These decision makers will vary from system to system but will likely include PBM administrators, pharmaceutical boards, P&T committees, drug purchasing groups, and utilization review managers. Many companies have responded to this change in key decision makers by forming national account management teams to develop and service large system-based accounts and by retraining their sales people to work within this new system.

The managed care environment has also greatly increased the role of nurse practitioners and physician assistants as targets for the sales efforts of pharmaceutical reps. Many states have increased the authority of these health care providers, and their role is expected to increase in the future. While there is variation in the degree of autonomy granted to nurse practitioners, they are currently authorized to write prescriptions in all but four states (13). Twenty-one states and the District of Columbia currently provide the authority to write prescriptions independently, and 15 of these states grant the authority to prescribe controlled substances (13). One recent survey suggests that both companies and their representatives are acknowledging the growing influence of nurse practitioners and physician assistants by focusing more training efforts on the role of these health care providers (14). As access to physicians continues to become more limited, the importance of nurse practitioners and physician assistants to the overall sales efforts of representatives will continue to increase.

While only a small percentage of specialized sales representatives may be responsible for handling these large accounts, many more will be working with physicians, pharmacists, and other key decision makers within the system. Therefore, all representatives will need to become familiar with the managed care accounts within their territory to work effectively in a team effort. They will also need to be aware of any contractual agreements made with organizations in their territory to be consistent with the terms of these contracts. In particular, pharmaceutical reps will require in-depth knowledge of local provider organizations, including information on key decision makers; basic organizational structure; and the organization's current use of outcomes research, clinical practice guidelines, and disease management programs. They will also require a growing familiarity with pharmacoeconomic research and methodology, such as cost-effectiveness studies and quality-of-life studies, and the ability to apply this information within a selling situation (5).

The influence of managed care and integrated health care systems has resulted in formularies that are increasingly restrictive. In this environment, product knowledge becomes particularly important. Key criteria used in assessing products for formulary approval are efficacy, safety, and cost (15). Consequently, sales representatives should be prepared to provide clinical data that demonstrate the therapeutic benefits and safety of their products, as well as pharmacoeconomic data that demonstrate cost-effectiveness. It is also becoming more important to differentiate products from competitors, as pharmacy and therapeutics committees are becoming more strict about adding what they see as duplicate products to the formulary.

To sell effectively within an integrated system, pharmaceutical representatives will need to define how each product should be positioned in terms of that system's:

- Product formulary, including the type of formulary used (open, closed, etc.), current formulary listings, and the mechanisms in place to move drugs on-formulary or to approve their off-formulary use
- Ongoing outcomes research and current outcomes data relating to given diseases or conditions
- Current use of clinical practice guidelines, including those developed by the provider system and those adapted from other sources
- Processes governing the development and updating of clinical practice guidelines, and the key players involved
- Current use of disease management programs and interest in additional programs or specific value-added services
- Contractual relationships with PBMs
- Current restrictions on access to health care professionals and any other restrictions on product promotions (5).

Armed with this knowledge, pharmaceutical reps will be in a stronger position to market their products successfully to integrated health care systems.

## NEW DIRECTIONS FOR PHARMACEUTICAL REPS

The pharmaceutical sales rep of the future is likely to be highly specialized but also will need to wear many different hats. Reps will be needed to act as consultants to a variety of health care providers and administrators, and their role as effective communicators will become increasingly critical as pharmaceutical companies expand into new areas, particularly disease management. Indeed, many companies have already moved to form specialized disease management reps, and more are expected to do so in the future. For example, Zeneca Pharmaceuticals recently formed a subsidiary (Stuart Disease Management Service), through which reps from Zeneca will be used to educate member physicians within managed care organizations with which the company has negotiated disease management contracts (16). Pfizer and Value Health have collaborated to form physician networks that will offer disease management services to managed care organizations (17). SmithKline Beecham's acquisition of DPS is expected to facilitate the development of its disease management programs (18). Also, Lilly has recently moved to reorganize into disease-based business units (19).

Pharmaceutical reps can expect to assume the more comprehensive role of service provider to the health care system within a disease management setting. These services will include the management of a variety of value-added programs for physicians, pharmacists, nurses, patients, and other health care providers and consumers, such as:

- Disease-oriented symposia and conferences
- Disease-oriented printed and audiovisual educational materials for health care professionals and patients
- In-service educational programs for physicians, pharmacists, and nurses
- Drug utilization review for the health care organization (7).

It is likely that specialized disease management reps will increase in numbers in the future.

Representatives specially trained in managed care are also likely to become more prevalent in the near future. Already, many companies have managed care representatives and teams, and many more are likely to do so. A recent survey by IMS America found that pharmaceutical representatives are highly rated by managed care executives in the area of improving formulary compliance (20). The effectiveness of pharmaceutical reps on managed care organizations is likely to continue to increase as reps become more educated and highly trained in this area. Today's managed care organizations are much more likely to provide access to pharmaceutical reps who are prepared to offer these purchasing groups more in the way of value-added services and beneficial economic data related to their product. By increasing their focus on the needs of these new customers, pharmaceutical reps will be in a better position to respond to the opportunity and potential to work both as consultants and partners within these organizations.

Another way in which pharmaceutical companies are responding to the changing health care environment is by employing more flex-time reps. These reps work on a part-time basis, typically have experience in the field, and are as well qualified as their full-time counterparts (21). Companies may also use these reps to promote older drugs which, while still profitable for companies, do not have the overall potential of newer products requiring a great deal of sales time. It is too soon to tell whether the use of flex-time reps will expand, but it is certain that pharmaceutical companies will continue experimenting with new ways to achieve the best results with their most effective marketing tool–the sales representative.

## CONCLUSION

As the health care industry in this country continues to evolve, the pharmaceutical sales force is likely to continue to experience change. One of the most important considerations for pharmaceutical reps will be the need to stay abreast of these changes through the continuation of their education. With the rapid transformation occurring in the industry, it is important to stay informed to communicate effectively with all health care providers and to be able to go beyond traditional product selling. More than ever before, reps will need to know how to interpret pharmacoeconomic studies, outcomes research, and quality-of-life studies to market their products successfully. Today's health care market offers many challenges for pharmaceutical reps, but it also provides new and exciting opportunities for representatives. The successful pharmaceutical sales representatives of the future will be those who are willing to continue their education to stay informed about current trends and issues. These include the movement toward disease management and integrated health care systems, which will continue to affect the industry into the next century.

## REFERENCES

1. Safian GR. Finding a new marketing Rx for pharmaceuticals. Public Relations J 1994;(Mar).

2. Introduction to managed healthcare. Roanoke, VA: Certified Medical Representatives Institute, 1995.

3. Marion Merrell Dow. Managed care digest: HMO edition. Kansas City, MO: Marion Merrell Dow, 1994.

4. Marion Merrell Dow. Managed care digest: PPO edition. Kansas City, MO: Marion Merrell Dow, 1994.

5. Advanced concepts in managed healthcare. Roanoke, VA: Certified Medical Representatives Institute, in press.

6. Tanouye E, Anders G. Drug industry takeovers mean more cost-cutting, less research spending. Wall Street J.

7. Total disease management. Roanoke, VA: Certified Medical Representatives Institute, 1995.

8. Walsh J. The sales manager's nightmare is really a wakeup call. Med Market Media 1994;29(May):22-30.

9. Number of reps drops by 700 in 1995. Pharm Rep 1995;(Mar).

10. Anon. Drug bulk buyers create need for select salespeople. Boston Globe.

11. Ross WR. Careers still flourish, but the rules have changed. Med Market Media 1994;29(Dec):20-6.

12. Hahn B. Employment outlook '94: more hard times. Pharm Exec 1994;14(June):64-74.

13. Changing roles of healthcare providers. Roanoke, VA: Certified Medical Representatives Institute, 1995.

14. Mittman DE, Yackeren TF, Hendrix P, Mirotznik G. Sales reps recognize value of nurse practitioners. Med Market Media 1994;29(July):52-4.

15. The formulary process–challenges and opportunities. Roanoke, VA: Certified Medical Representatives Institute, 1995.

16. Anon. Schering-Plough would partner with other drug companies to buy PBM; disease management contracts in place with 62 managed care customers. FDC Rep–Pink Sheet 1994;56(28):4.

17. Anon. Pfizer/Value Health $100 mil. joint venture will establish physician networks for disease management; firms enter product support, formulary agreements. FDC Rep–Pink Sheet 1994;56(19):13-4.

18. Anon. SmithKline Beecham is going into PBM business via $2.3 bil. purchase of DPS: HMO niche of business may offer control advantage compared to Medco/PAID. FDC Rep–Pink Sheet 1994;56(19):10-2.

19. Anon. Lilly reorganization into disease-based business units advances firm toward systems-oriented sales model; focus on internal medicine, endocrinology, CNS. FDC Rep–Pink Sheet 1994;56(29):9.

20. Anon. Sales forces may be undervalued as tools. FDC Rep–Pink Sheet 1994;56(41):5.

21. Castagnoli WG. Business prospects promising for freelance field forces. Med Market Media 1994;29(Aug):136-9.

# Pharmaceutical Marketing Research: A Blueprint for the Future

Lea Prevel Katsanis
Mrugank V. Thakor

## INTRODUCTION

The escalating pace of change in the health care industry that has been motivated by concern over rising costs has major implications for health professionals, pharmaceutical firms, and patients. This concern has been fueled by the high proportion of the GNP dedicated to health care related expenses in the U.S. relative to other industrialized countries, the large number of Americans without health coverage, and rising health insurance premiums for middle-class families. While there are undoubtedly multiple underlying causes of the problems, the popular and business presses have focused on the profits made by insurers and pharmaceutical firms. For instance, a recent cover story in *Fortune* highlighted the repeated price increases of major drugs and the relationship between these hikes and the steady uptrend in pharmaceutical firm profits (1).

Among the most significant health care developments in recent years has been the growth of health maintenance organizations with a mandate to use buying efficiencies to control costs. Their interest in substituting

Lea Prevel Katsanis, Ph.D., is Assistant Professor of Marketing in the Faculty of Commerce and Administration at Concordia University, 1455 de Maisonneuve Boulevard West, Montreal, Quebec, Canada H3G 1M8. Mrugank V. Thakor, Ph.D., is Assistant Professor of Marketing in the Faculty of Commerce and Administration at Concordia University.

[Haworth co-indexing entry note]: "Pharmaceutical Marketing Research: A Blueprint for the Future." Katsanis, Lea Prevel and Mrugank V. Thakor. Co-published simultaneously in *Journal of Pharmaceutical Marketing & Management* (Pharmaceutical Products Press, an imprint of The Haworth Press, Inc.) Vol. 10, No. 4, 1996, pp. 251-267; and: *Pharmaceutical Marketing in the 21st Century* (ed: Mickey C. Smith) Pharmaceutical Products Press, an imprint of The Haworth Press, Inc., 1996, pp. 251-265. Single or multiple copies of this article are available from The Haworth Document Delivery Service [1-800-342-9678, 9:00 a.m. - 5:00 p.m. (EST)].

cheaper drugs for more expensive ones where at all possible and negotiating the lowest possible prices puts them in direct conflict with the interests of pharmaceutical companies (2). However, the latter have recognized these emerging realities and have moved to integrate vertically by acquiring both HMOs and pharmaceutical benefit management companies (e.g., Merck and Medco, SmithKline Beecham and DPS, Eli Lilly and PCS) (3). Despite the many unique features of the health care environment, such as the critical nature of products that affect patients' health and lives, these acquisitions appear to mirror changes other industries have undergone. Although the parallels are far from exact, the airline and ocean shipping industries are two others where the delivery of value to the customer includes both a large service component–as does health care–as well as powerful channel representatives similar to HMOs (consolidators). Interestingly, these industries also responded to the emergence of influential channel intermediaries by integrating vertically, with mixed results. Drawing inferences from these imperfect analogies, it appears that acquiring HMOs and PBMs may not be the complete answer and that there may be no substitute for "owning" the customer with the help of differentiated drugs and direct-to-consumer promotion. The changing landscape of the health care industry of which these new alliances are a part seems to demand major rethinking of conventional strategic assumptions as well as of the kind of marketing research that has been done in the past. With this in mind, the authors set out to assess the kinds of research that has recently been published and then to establish some guidelines regarding the kind of research likely to be required in the future. The methodology employed and the findings uncovered are reported below.

## STUDY METHODOLOGY

The methodology used in this study was twofold: a content analysis of the *Journal of Pharmaceutical Marketing & Management* over a 5-year time frame from 1990 to 1994 to evaluate past trends in pharmaceutical marketing research and personal telephone interviews using a convenience sample consisting of both pharmaceutical marketing research executives from leading pharmaceutical companies and senior consultants from major custom market research houses specializing in pharmaceutical research. This dual research method was employed to determine the relevance of the topics that have traditionally been researched over the past five years, as well as to identify topics of future interest.

The *Journal of Pharmaceutical Marketing & Management* was chosen for the content analysis because it is devoted solely to the study of the pharmaceutical industry. To some extent, it can be considered a bellwether for the topics of interest to both practitioners and scholars with a strong interest in the pharmaceutical industry.

With respect to the telephone interviews, it was believed that both internal marketing research executives and senior consultants needed to be contacted, as congruence on topic areas could be measured by comparison. Additionally, the general business literature was examined through ABI-Inform to identify potential topics of importance to these industry members. Key informants were also used prior to conducting these interviews to verify the topic areas. Respondents were provided with various topic areas and asked to rate them in terms of importance to the industry. This data was then used to generate discussion on the various types of research that could be required.

This study is limited both by the sample size and the method of sample selection. However, due to the homogeneity of the industry and the small number of individuals who specialize in pharmaceutical market research, it was believed that the importance of the findings, even for a small sample, outweighed some of the limitations. Also, through triangulation of data sources, the authors feel that additional support can be given to the findings (4).

## CONTENT ANALYSIS: THE KEY TOPIC AREA REVIEW

The review of key topics revealed the following in order of magnitude: patients and pharmacists, 36 articles each; promotion, 9 articles; physicians and organizational research, 8 articles each; and products, 3 articles, for a total of 100 articles over the 5-year period. Each topic area is covered in detail below.

### Patients

In this topic area, four general areas of research emerged: (1) consumer attitudes, profiles and behavior (31% of articles); (2) pharmacy patronage/shopping habits (28% of articles); (3) product usage (22% of articles); and (4) patient sources of information (19% of articles). There were 36 articles in total, and interest in this area has remained constant over the 5-year period. However, the topics of increasing interest are consumer profiling and consumer sources of information. The sample types studied were varied, but the greatest emphasis was placed on examining the general population, with the elderly/senior population being the next largest demographic group to be examined. The remainder of the articles dealt with either students or families or were theoretical in nature.

Those articles that took a product focus were equally divided between OTC and prescription products and were the majority. These were followed by generics and then health and beauty aids. Pharmacists were the key professional group examined, while only one article dealt with physician issues. The content of each topic area is summarized below, with a focus on the studies of greatest importance to the area.

*Consumer Profiles, Attitudes, and Behavior*

One of the major subjects covered is that of generic consumers: who they are, how they respond to advertising, and what their attitudes are in general toward these drugs. These studies are important, as more and more products are coming off patent and as price sensitive consumers are seeking out the best prices for prescription drugs. This area will become even more important as large managed health care groups begin to purchase their own drugs for distribution to those covered by their plans.

Strutton, Pelton, and Lumpkin profiled the "generic-prone" consumer in the OTC domain (5). Perri and Wolfgang examined changes in behavior after a direct-to-consumer advertising campaign focusing on generic prescription medications (6).

*Pharmacy Patronage/Shopping Habits*

This area of the research concentrated on why consumers purchase their prescription and OTC drugs in specific locations or in a certain manner. Given the current interest in mail-order pharmacies and managed health care plans, two studies were of particular interest in this category. Carroll and Fincham examined the elderly's views of mail order and found that the primary motivator for mail-order usage is price rather than convenience (7). Donehew found that shopping patterns changed very little for OTC drugs after patients became members of a managed health care plan (8).

*Product Usage*

This topic area has declined in interest over the last five years, possibly as a result of an increase in the amount of custom research available to companies directly, as well as for competitive reasons. However, one key area of the research focused on the intended use of nonprescription drugs with respect to risk perception (9).

*Sources of Information*

This area of research has been gradually increasing in interest since 1989, with three studies appearing in 1994 alone. Part of the reason for this interest is that with the overwhelming amount of advertising in both the prescription and nonprescription drug areas and the changing role of health care professionals, consumers are faced with multiple sources of information about their drugs. One major area of importance is that of where and how consumers receive product information. Portner and Smith discovered that formal sources (physicians and pharmacists) were the most accurate but least convenient, while informal sources, such as family and TV, were less accurate but more convenient (10). Eppright and Cunningham found that older consumers were more interested in using product ingredient and professional information, while younger consumers relied on brand name, price, and the general media (11).

## *Pharmacists*

This has been one of the major areas of research interest for authors publishing in this journal. A total of 36 articles have appeared on aspects of this topic over the last 5 years. This level of interest is understandable in view of the key role pharmacists have historically played in the distribution of both OTC and prescription drugs.

Although many different themes are represented in the body of research on pharmacists, the principal ones are: (1) factors affecting pharmacists' (drug) product choices and merchandising decisions, including those related to generics, 25%; (2) pharmacists' job-and career-related attitudes and behaviors, such as satisfaction, commitment, role perceptions, 28%; (3) pharmacy operations, strategic planning, and performance, 22%; and (4) other, including pharmacists' consulting and prescribing behavior, 25%.

The pattern of publication of papers in these areas is such that interest appears to shift from one area to another every few years. For instance, the topic area relating to how choices between drugs are made by pharmacists and how merchandising decisions are made enjoyed more popularity in the beginning of this decade. Between 1990 and 1992, a total of seven articles were published relating to this topic, but only two were published in the years 1993 and 1994, one of which used a sample of Finnish pharmacists. This is particularly surprising in light of the fact that the issue of generic substitution remains at least as relevant today as in earlier years.

An interesting diversity of samples was evident; subjects were comprised of independent pharmacists, pharmacists employed by chains, staff pharmacists employed by hospitals, hospital administrators, chain store managers, and patients.

*Factors Affecting Pharmacists' Drug Product Choices*

This subarea of research can be characterized by the degree of generality of the studies in terms of the products considered: generic vs. branded drugs or drugs in general. In the first category, Nagasawa, Smith, Monk, and Banahan used cluster analysis to segment and profile retail pharmacists based on likelihood of substituting generics for 17 brand-name products (12). In the same vein, Holmes and Dennison sought to explain student pharmacists' decisions to recommend generic rather than branded products (13). Holmes and Dennison found that elements of perceived risk significantly affected the recommendations made. Researchers have also looked at pharmacists' drug choice decisions in a more basic and theoretically grounded manner to ascertain how pharmacists determine recommendation and stocking policies. Emmerton and Benrimoj, when looking at nonprescription products, found that product formulation and probability of successful self-use had the strongest effects on pharmacists' recommendations (14).

*Pharmacists' Job-and Career-Related Attitudes and Behaviors*

Among the pharmacist attitudes considered by the ten articles in this area are overall job satisfaction, satisfaction with the supervisor, and career commitment. Among those who focused on elements of pharmacists' satisfaction, Kozma and colleagues found that the implementing of new programs by pharmacies produced small but significant increases in pharmacists' job satisfaction (15). Gubbins and Rascati found that when the area supervisor in chain stores was not a pharmacist, this had a significant negative effect on pharmacists' satisfaction with the supervisor (16).

Undoubtedly motivated by the high costs associated with turnover, researchers have also considered pharmacists' career intentions. Reid, Johnson, and Robertson investigated factors influencing the career commitment of pharmacists and found that personal fulfillment and achievement, recognition by supervisors, and future prospects for financial security were among the more important explanatory variables (17).

*Pharmacy Operations, Strategic Planning, and Performance*

Several of the eight articles in this area have looked at strategic issues from the standpoint of institutional pharmacy administrators. Harrison and Bootman point out that, despite its importance to institutional pharmacies, strategic planning is grossly underresearched at this level (18). Birdwell,

Sirdeshmukh, and Pathak surveyed hospital pharmacy directors and concluded that a model of environmental analysis was useful to respondents in assessing threats and opportunities facing them (19). Responding to their own call for research in this area, Harrison and Bootman examined the extent and quality of strategic planning practice by institutional pharmacy directors (20). Their findings were encouraging in that the majority of respondents reported using strategic planning and rated pharmacy performance in several areas higher than those who did not use strategic planning.

## Pharmacists' Consulting and Prescribing Behavior

Researchers have shown considerable interest in the pharmacist's role as a counselor and information provider to patients, relative to the role as product provider, as evidenced by the eight articles on this topic. Several studies have used Florida pharmacists as subjects, in view of their limited ability to prescribe without physician guidance. Eng and colleagues used trained shoppers in Florida and found that pharmacists did not elicit general health and medical history information from patients very well but were conscientious in complying with legal requirements regarding labeling and quantity limitations (21).

In a more general context, a Vancouver study found that pharmacists overestimated their own importance as monitors of compliance and information providers relative to the perceptions of patients and physicians, suggesting a need for pharmacists to educate others about their capabilities (22). These empirical studies complement well a recent article that discusses pharmacists' evolving legal liability in two areas: side effects of therapy and interactions with other drugs (23).

## Products

While potentially extremely important, the products area has generated little research appearing in this journal. Possibly this is because most of such research is done on a proprietary basis. An interesting effort to consider the role of the product life cycle concept as a planning tool was undertaken by Jernigan and colleagues (24). They described the 15-year trends of new prescription volumes of some drug products introduced between 1963 and 1972.

## Firms

There were a total of six articles in this area. Somewhat surprisingly, in view of the current changes in the U.S. health care industry, only one of these articles considered the effect of the growing importance of managed health care organizations on the pharmaceutical industry (25). The authors found that managed health care plans were expected to cover 45% of all outpatient prescriptions in 5 years and about 70% in 10 years. The shift to managed health care was also expected to lead to a greater emphasis on pharmacoeconomics.

Ross and Nydick discuss within the context of Sterling Drugs' efforts to license new drugs for the treatment of cancer the use of the Analytic Hierarchy Process (26). The AHP allows for explicit evaluation of criteria which can be scientific, business, or strategic. This appears to be a viable and interesting approach to organizational decision making.

### Promotion

Promotion of pharmaceuticals has traditionally been an area of importance for both practitioners and academics alike, and with direct-to-consumer advertising as part of the marketing mix, research has become a bit more interesting. However, most of this research is done at the firm/consultant level due to confidentiality considerations, and not much has appeared in academic journals.

Over the past five years, nine articles have appeared in this area, with slightly over half of these written since 1992. Topics in this area are diverse, but patient portrayal–how patients are portrayed in advertising and what implications this has for them–is the primary topic of interest to researchers.

Rallapalli, Smith, and Stone examined the social portrayal of individuals in OTC magazine advertisements and found that it did not differ from their portrayal in other forms of advertising (27). However, OTC magazine ads tend to portray racial and ethnic minorities less frequently. Ho and Smith found that the elderly are underrepresented in television OTC drug advertisements, and this may affect their role and image adversely (28).

### Physicians

The category of physician research was one of the smallest, with eight articles. The studies concerned themselves with product switching and advertising techniques (sources of information). The key study in this area was that of Madhavan and Gore, which examined physicians' attitudes toward the switching of drugs from prescription to OTC status (29). Overall, physicians had negative attitudes toward switching and self-medication, as well as the prescribing of switched drug products.

Another interesting article was that of Engle, which concerned the impact of single-advertiser publications on physicians' perceptions (30). The results obtained suggest that the reading of at least one company-sponsored vehicle had a substantial impact on physicians' perceptions of the sponsoring company and on the frequency with which they expected to prescribe. This study has significant implications for pharmaceutical companies, given that much of their promotional budgets are spent on multi-sponsorship vehicles and journal advertising.

## *KEY FINDINGS–INDUSTRY INTERVIEWS*

Twenty pharmaceutical marketing research executives and market research consultants were asked to rank seven topic areas–managed care, patient outcomes, changing role of the physician, changing role of the pharmacist, advertising and promotion testing, marketing organization strategies, and pricing–based on whether they considered a research topic of great importance or of lesser importance. In order of greatest importance to least importance, the topics were rated as follows: patient outcomes, managed care, pricing, marketing organizational structure, changing role of the physician, changing role of the pharmacist, and advertising and promotional strategies.

It is important to note that respondents believe that most of these topics are closely interrelated and that future research needs to address these interrelationships. For example, patient outcomes research will determine the prices that both managed care units and patients may be willing to pay for drugs. The fact that patient outcomes are being considered at all puts the patient at the center of any research that is to be conducted in the future. In fact, the patient emphasis will affect product choices based on price as well as the menu of services that managed care groups will offer (e.g., choice of physicians) to patients.

Additionally, according to respondents, the future of pharmacists and physicians seems to be affiliation with large managed care units as opposed to the traditional model of community pharmacies and solo practitioners. Their role within these managed care units, perhaps as gatekeepers and decision makers, will affect how pharmaceutical products are promoted and who the "real" customer will be. This, in turn, affects the marketing organizational strategy chosen by a pharmaceutical company that will best meet this changing promotional and customer environment.

There seems to be a general consensus among respondents that issues in the industry are a moving target. It is extremely difficult in the current environment to set a research agenda. The topics covered as part of this research were acknowledged as important, but respondents interviewed believe that issues will need to unfold further before they feel completely comfortable formulating a blueprint for the future.

### Patient Outcomes Research

This was by far the most important area identified by respondents, both on the industry and supplier sides. In fact, there were few, if any, differences between them in terms of the critical need for research on this topic.

The basic need for research seems to be how a company can measure patient outcomes. All respondents reported that industry, government, and managed care units appear to be using different pharmacoeconomic models. For example, some are based on cost-benefit analysis; others are based on quality of life years. However, there is no consensus on which is the best way to measure patient outcomes, and developing a model for measurement will be a critical area for research.

Several respondents suggested that market researchers develop database marketing systems in conjunction with clinical trials (post-Phase 3; pre-Phase 4) that would represent real-life tracking data based on therapeutic class. Another respondent noted that the outcomes will differ not only by therapeutic class but also by the seriousness of the disease. For example, cardiovascular drugs for arrhythmias may have a different outcome path from NSAIDs for arthritis.

Research in this area is needed to determine who the decision makers are. As one respondent reported: "Also important is who the key decision maker will be–in the case of arthritis, it may be the P & T Committee at a managed care unit; in the case of cardiology, it may be the physician."

One issue all respondents agreed on was that the research must be patient driven; it must consider the needs and concerns of patients, as inevitably, they will be paying the final prices for drugs. Some specific topics mentioned by respondents included:

1. How much will patients, as well as managed care units, be willing to pay for products based on the perceived therapeutic outcome for them?
2. Will patients pay more for drugs they perceive to offer higher quality? How is product quality factored into the cost/price equation when considering patient outcomes?

One respondent was quite eloquent on the need for market researchers to be involved in this area: "A real opportunity exists for market researchers in this area . . . the industry doesn't know what patients think, only what doctors tell them. We need to hear the voice of the patient."

Finally, one industry respondent pointed out the need for research that documents how drugs act to prevent serious disease and thus reduce the overall cost of health care.

## Managed Care

This topic area generated a host of potential areas for research, primarily because, according to one respondent, "No one really knows what questions we should be asking these large organizations." However, despite this concern, respondents on both the industry and the supplier sides generated a variety of potential research topics for consideration:

1.  What are the key concerns of managed care providers? Who do they consider to be their key customers and how can pharmaceutical companies assist them in conducting their business? One industry executive commented: "Managed care groups will be one of our key target markets in the future, and we need to plan and analyze their needs."
2.  How do patients perceive the quality of treatment they receive from managed health care providers? Can pharmaceutical companies help managed health care providers give quality care?
3.  How will managed care groups affect the insurance industry? Are insurance companies competing already, and if not, what strategies will they adopt to enter this market? Will pharmaceutical companies buy insurance companies and use them as a way of entering the managed care business? As one consultant put it, "Right now, insurance companies are just bankers . . . but we expect this to change very soon."

## Pricing

As stated earlier, this area of potential research is directly related to patient outcomes research. There were two general areas of potential research mentioned by both industry and suppliers: one concerns pricing sensitivity and establishing value in pricing strategy, and the other concerns pricing methods and negotiating strategies with large managed care providers and the government.

In the area of establishing value, two key areas of potential research emerged:

1.  How do pharmaceutical companies establish value for their products given the multiple customers they will have to address, including managed care units, the government, and patients?

2. How do we measure pricing sensitivity with respect to patients? Where do patients enter the pricing equation?
3. What strategies can a pharmaceutical company use to convince managed care units of continued value vis à vis pricing?

With respect to pricing methods and negotiating strategies, two respondents noted that pricing research must combine economic modeling with outcomes research. One topic area of great interest was that of negotiating strategy, the strategies firms can use to ensure that their products appear on managed care formularies.

### Marketing Organization Strategies

While interest in this area was quite high, the scope of the topics suggested was significantly narrower than for other topic areas. This is possibly because certain organizational trends in general have emerged that pharmaceutical organizations have already implemented. Both industry researchers and suppliers identified three key topic areas for research: regionalization, globalization, and business intelligence units.

1. Are regional marketing units an effective organizational design for pharmaceutical companies, given the nature of the business, and how has this organizational structure affected the implementation of marketing strategy? One consultant said: "When I asked my client why they had reorganized into regional marketing units, he said with some embarrassment that it was because everyone else was doing it."

There seems to be some concern that the regional approach, which works in consumer goods firms, may not be the most appropriate approach for the pharmaceutical industry, and it needs to be studied more closely.

2. Some large multinational firms have strong central headquarters. How can this organizational structure be best managed globally?
3. What is the importance of business intelligence units within pharmaceutical companies, and how will this change the role of the traditional market researcher within this environment?

One industry researcher commented that traditional market researchers may be "in jeopardy of becoming a dinosaur" unless they carve a new role for themselves. They are now being replaced by business intelligence managers or outcomes research managers in some large multinational companies. The future of their role needs further examination.

## Changing Role of the Physician

When compared to other topics, this area was of somewhat lesser priority because a great deal of quality research about physicians already exists. One respondent noted that "we pretty much know everything we need to know about doctors." When probed further, however, several respondents generated several important areas for future research:

1. How has managed care changed the physician's perception of himself or herself (e.g., loss of control)?
2. What is the new decision-making role of the physician within the managed care context?
3. How do we provide customer service to physicians given their reduced role in the prescribing decision?

It is clear from the data that, despite lower priority, the physician remains a key individual in the mix.

## Changing Role of the Pharmacist

Respondents were also satisfied with the research to date on pharmacists because of the considerable number and scope of the studies already available. Several respondents generated the following research topics:

1. How much power will pharmacists have in a managed care setting? What will their decision-making role be in this setting?
2. What should the pharmacist's role be in assisting with patient compliance and patient education?
3. What will the impact of mail-order pharmacies such as Medco—which has the force of a major multinational company backing it–be on chain store pharmacies and community pharmacies?

The primary concern of respondents on this topic is the new relationship between the pharmacist and the managed health care unit, whether the pharmacist is employed by a large chain or works within a managed care setting.

## Advertising and Promotion Research

This last topic area was not perceived to be as critical as others mentioned by respondents. This is seen as "tactical" versus "strategic" research and tends to be very situation specific. There was little topic agreement among respondents regarding this area. However, some potential research priorities generated by those with an interest in this area were:

1. What is the role of the pharmaceutical company's promotion and advertising in patient education about disease prevention and treatment?
2. What selling approach is most effective in dealing with managed care units? Who are the key decision makers, and how many individuals need to be seen in each unit to have the maximum selling impact (e.g., administrators, physicians, pharmacists, nurses, etc.)?
3. How do we value the service of sales representatives given changes in the marketing organization (e.g., regional marketing units)? How do physicians and others respond to this organizational change?
4. Not enough is currently known about how direct-to-consumer advertising works and whether it works.
5. What standard methodology should be used to test promotional materials, whether they are journal ads or detailing aids?

It would appear from the data that the bulk of this type of research will continue to be conducted at the firm level as a result of the need for confidentiality.

## IMPLICATIONS OF RESEARCH

When the research findings from both the content analysis and primary research are examined, it is apparent that certain changes are indicated in the topics to be studied, whether one is an academic researcher or a researcher who works for multinationals or market research consultants. It is evident that patient-level research must be refocused to outcomes and pricing versus the traditional consumer behavior and product research emphasis. Levels of research in the areas of advertising and promotion strategy, as well as product research, seem to be in keeping with the current interest expressed in them. The changing roles of the physician and the pharmacist, given the managed care setting, require a refocusing of traditional academic and practitioner research. This shift in emphasis will provide academic researchers with ample opportunities for studies that will be of use to the pharmaceutical industry. These researchers already have a wealth of experience in studying these two professional groups in their traditional roles, as evidenced by the content analysis presented in this study.

The area of patient outcomes is clearly a priority, and one which will likely be handled at the industry level by multinational firms and market research consultants in conjunction with government and other health professionals. However, academic marketing researchers can make a contribution here, particularly with the creation of models and the testing of those models. It will be important to have an unbiased view when examining the various alternatives that will be proposed by different constituencies.

The study of managed care organizations is one in which academic researchers can make a particularly strong contribution. Through survey research, much data can be obtained from these organizations and provided to practitioners.

Marketing organizational structure can be studied by academic researchers through case studies and qualitative methodologies. There is much to understand about how different structures affect marketing strategy within pharmaceutical firms.

Pricing analysis, particularly pricing sensitivity, is another research area in which strong contributions can be made. Academic marketing researchers have particular expertise in this field, and research energy should be devoted here, specifically focusing on pharmaceutical pricing.

Finally, it is important to note that the roles of both market research consultants and industry market researchers are rapidly changing: in the first instance, to a consultative versus data-collecting role and in the second instance, to a more strategic intelligence role.

## CONCLUSIONS

Over the next five years and into the 21st century, major changes are under way in the pharmaceutical industry. It will be important for all those interested and concerned about the industry to provide high quality and relevant research for the challenges ahead. Research must move more quickly and respond to those challenges. The authors believe that all market researchers are in a position to make major contributions to the future of this vital industry.

## REFERENCES

1. O'Reilly B. Drugmakers under attack. Fortune 1991;(Jul 29):48.
2. Ross WR. The coming battle over marketing turf. Med Market Media 1994;29(June):32-6.

3. Seiden CJ. Landmines threaten industry responses to managed care. Med Market Media 1994;29(Oct):68-70.

4. Miles MB, Huberman AM. Qualitative data analysis–a sourcebook of new methods. Newbury Park, CA: Sage Publications, 1984.

5. Strutton D, Pelton LE, Lumpkin JR. Profiling the generic-prone consumer: implications for the promotion of generic and branded OTC medications. J Pharm Market Manage 1994;8(2):3-25.

6. Perri M, Wolfgang AP. Consumers' cognitive and behavioral responses to a health care advertising campaign. J Pharm Market Manage 1992;6(3):75-88.

7. Carroll NV, Fincham JE. Elderly consumers' views of community and mail-order pharmacies. J Pharm Market Manage 1992;6(3):3-32.

8. Donehew GR. Pharmacy products shopping patterns of members before and after joining a large managed health care plan: a pilot study. J Pharm Market Manage 1992;6(3):21-32.

9. Charupatanapong N, Rascati KL. An analysis of consumers' risk perceptions of their self-medication practices. J Pharm Market Manage 1991;5(4):53-78.

10. Portner TS, Smith MC. College students' perceptions of OTC information source characteristics. J Pharm Market Manage 1994;8(1):161-85.

11. Eppright DR, Cunningham ICM. Demographic and health locus of control influences on nonprescription drug information use expectations. J Pharm Market Manage 1994;8(3):29-47.

12. Nagasawa M, Smith MC, Monk MR, Banahan BF III. Profiling retail pharmacist segments identified with respect to generic substitution. J Pharm Market Manage 1992;6(4):33-52.

13. Holmes JH, Dennison KM. Student pharmacists' perceptions of generic and branded drugs. J Pharm Market Manage 1992;6(4):71-83.

14. Emmerton LM, Benrimoj SI. Influences on pharmacists' stocking and recommendation of nonprescription products. J Pharm Market Manage 1991;5(3):37-50.

15. Kozma CM, Hirsch JD, Mackowiak J, Bloise A, Gagnon JP. Implementing a pharmacy services program: impact on pharmacists' job satisfaction. J Pharm Market Manage 1993;7(4):25-40.

16. Gubbins TV, Rascati KL. Satisfaction with management and overall job satisfaction of Texas chain store pharmacists. J Pharm Market Manage 1992;6(3):59-74.

17. Ried LD, Johnson RE, Robertson N. Factors associated with pharmacists' career commitment. J Pharm Market Manage 1990;5(1):45-67.

18. Harrison DL, Bootman JL. Strategic planning for institutional pharmacy administrators. J Pharm Market Manage 1990;5(1):29-43.

19. Birdwell SW, Sirdeshmukh D, Pathak DS. Environmental analysis in hospital pharmacy: assessing threats and opportunities. J Pharm Market Manage 1990;4(4):41-58.

20. Harrison DL, Bootman JL. Strategic planning by institutional pharmacy administrators. J Pharm Market Manage 1994;8(2):73-96.

21. Eng HJ, Bulfer BA, Doering PL, Kimberlin CL. Assessment of the Florida Pharmacist Self-Care Consultant Law using a trained shopper method. J Pharm Market Manage 1991;5(4):27-52.

22. Stratton TP, Stewart EE. The role of the community pharmacist in providing drug and health information: a pilot survey among the public, physicians, and pharmacists. J Pharm Market Manage 1991;5(4):3-26.

23. Hall M, Honey W. The evolving legal responsibility of the pharmacist. J Pharm Market Manage 1994;8(2):27-41.

24. Jernigan JM, Smith MC, Banahan BF, Juergens JP. Descriptive analysis of the 15-year product life cycles of a sample of pharmaceutical products. J Pharm Market Manage 1991;6(1):3-36.

25. Summers KH, Gumbhir AK. The expected impact of managed health care organizations on the research-intensive U.S. pharmaceutical industry. J Pharm Market Manage 1991;5(3):65-77.

26. Ross ME, Nydick RL. Structuring the selection process of licensing candidates in the pharmaceutical industry using the Analytic Hierarchy Process. J Pharm Market Manage 1994;8(1):21-36.

27. Rallapalli KC, Smith MC, Stone GW. The social portrayal of people in OTC drug advertising: a content analysis of magazine advertisements. J Pharm Market Manage 1994;8(2):111-26.

28. Ho FN, Smith MC. Portrayal of the elderly in over-the-counter drug television advertisements. J Pharm Market Manage 1992;6(4):21-31.

29. Madhavan S, Gore P. A multidimensional analysis of physicians' perceptions of Rx-to-OTC switched drug products. J Pharm Market Manage 1994;8(3):3-28.

30. Engle RL. The impact of a single-advertiser publication on physicians' perceptions and expected prescribing behavior. J Pharm Market Manage 1994;8(1):37-54.

# A Look at the Pharmaceutical Industry in the 21st Century

## Stephen C. Chappell

### INTRODUCTION

Contemplating the structure of the pharmaceutical industry in the 21st century would have been a relatively simple task if one had been asked to do so ten years ago, or even five years ago. A statement on the order of "Please refer to the 1980s," with some minor modifications, would have addressed the subject more than adequately.

But the first half of the current decade has been characterized much more by revolution than evolution in the industry, and the fruits of that revolutionary process appear likely to be the bricks and mortar that will form the bulk of the structure of the industry in the 21st century. In short, "what's past is prologue" doesn't seem to apply. It is, instead, what has come to be called the "new reality" upon which an assessment of the industry in the next century must be based.

### THE NEW REALITY

The 1980s were glory years for the pharmaceutical industry, spurred by major growth in antiulcerants, antibiotics, new cardiovascular agents, and the first of the biotechnology products. But 1992 and 1993 brought a new

---

Stephen C. Chappell, Esq., is Senior Vice President at IMS International, 660 West Germantown Pike, Plymouth Meeting, PA 19462-0905.

[Haworth co-indexing entry note]: "A Look at the Pharmaceutical Industry in the 21st Century." Chappell, Stephen C. Co-published simultaneously in *Journal of Pharmaceutical Marketing & Management* (Pharmaceutical Products Press, an imprint of The Haworth Press, Inc.) Vol. 10, No. 4, 1996, pp. 269-283; and: *Pharmaceutical Marketing in the 21st Century* (ed: Mickey C. Smith) Pharmaceutical Products Press, an imprint of The Haworth Press, Inc., 1996, pp. 269-283. Single or multiple copies of this article are available from The Haworth Document Delivery Service [1-800-342-9678, 9:00 a.m. - 5:00 p.m. (EST)].

reality to the industry. Although the new reality appeared with a rush, in retrospect, the pressures had been building for some time.

Health care budgets had been growing beyond acceptable limits. While governments, generally the payers for health care (outside the United States), had been reluctant to interfere with health benefit schemes, they found that demand was increasing at a geometric rate, while they could afford to increase health care budgets only at an arithmetic rate. Primary factors in the growth of demand and costs were the aging of the population in the industrialized countries, increased health care coverage, the advent of high-technology products, growth in consumer demands, and anti-quated health care systems.

In the face of these escalating health care costs, governments in Europe and Japan looked for areas where costs could be easily cut, and pharmaceuticals were quickly identified. While drugs represent a comparatively small share of overall health care costs, these costs–unlike costs in other segments of health care–are discrete, easily identified, and easily quantified. These efforts at drug cost containment took many forms: price and profit controls, access and reimbursement controls through "de-listings," positive and negative reimbursement lists, reference pricing, and pressures on patients via fixed prescription charges and percentage copayments. While much of the targeting had been on the supply side, efforts have been seen as well to control the demand side in the form of fixed prescribing budgets for physicians, the supplying of detailed prescribing data, prescribing guidelines, and treatment protocols.

The general inability of the industry to obtain sought-after prices for newly introduced products, to raise prices, or even to maintain prices in many countries outside the U.S. resulted in increased pressures for financial return in the U.S., essentially the only "free market" among the major pharmaceutical markets. As one element of generating that return, the industry effected price increases in the U.S. that rode above standard measures such as PPI or CPI. Another element was the changing of mix, or the replacing of older drugs with newer, more effective, but more expensive drugs.

Although the purpose of price increases in the U.S. was to offset the lack of sufficient return elsewhere, the sword was double-edged. These increases became the focus of attention by legislators and, through legislators and others, the public. The need for revenues and profits to reinvest in research and development of new compounds to better control or cure diseases (and, ultimately, to lower the costs of health care by so doing) was, and continues to be, an argument that many refuse to hear. Additionally, the price disparities between branded and generic drugs became even more pronounced, opening the door even wider to successful generic competition once the patents of the brands expired. Ultimately, political and public opposition to the pricing and price increase policies of the brand-name sector of the U.S. industry became so severe as to cause most brand companies to pledge to keep post-1992 percentage price increases to CPI rates, or less than half of pre-1992 levels of increase.

Other pressures on revenue and profit began to build. Federal legislation resulted in the mandating of substantial price discounts, or rebates, from manufacturers whose products were reimbursed by state Medicaid programs. Third-party payers increasingly looked to formulary systems to contain costs and mandated with more frequency the prescribing or dispensing of generics where available. Mail-order pharmacy became more of a factor in the market. Here, too, quantity discounts were demanded of the manufacturer. The formation of buying alliances among other prescription dispensers was noted. Doctors began to feel more pressure to prescribe economically.

Price competition among different branded products, previously not a factor, became a serious issue. As price, rather than more traditional product claims, became a major factor in the decision as to which product(s) in a therapy class a third-party payer would place on its formulary, or reimburse, patent-protected products in certain categories began competing with each other on the basis of price. As a result, the advantage of having a distinct and nonduplicated drug lessened considerably.

The above and other factors contributed to a sudden and severe slowdown in sales and profits in 1992-1993 for virtually every major drug company. Along with this abrupt change, R&D pipelines, the lifeblood of the pharmaceutical business, were growing empty.

Further results of the new reality were massive declines in the stock prices of drug companies as Wall Street reassessed their value. In addition, the industry's image continued to be sullied by attacks from the government and a continuing public perception of excessive pricing and price increases.

Layered on top of all of the above was the prospect of the Clinton Plan.

## THE CLINTON PLAN

In retrospect, the Clinton health care reform initiative (American Health Security Act) was a remarkable piece of nonlegislation, at least with respect to its impact on the U.S. pharmaceutical industry. While the Clinton Plan never saw the light of day as enacted legislation, the U.S. industry responded as though the plan's provisions regarding drugs and drug utilization would be set in place. In effect, the industry was "out in front" of an event that didn't occur.

The more significant aspects of the Clinton Plan for the drug industry were:

- The concept of managed care or managed competition would be a basic modality in the provision of and the payment for health care.
- An outpatient prescription drug benefit for Medicare patients which would provide reimbursement for drug expenditures to those of the elderly who had no prescription drug coverage. If a branded drug was used for these patients, the manufacturer would be required to rebate Medicare for roughly 17% of the drug's average trade price.
- The Medicare benefit would cover only generics if a generic drug were available.
- Physicians and pharmacists might need prior approval for the prescribing or dispensing of certain pharmaceuticals if the Secretary of Health and Human Services had determined that these medications were not cost-effective. Criteria were provided in the plan for the determination of excessive or inappropriate drug prices: (1) prices of other drugs in the same therapeutic category, (2) costs of production, (3) prices in other comparable countries, and (4) other relevant factors. None of these criteria, of course, provides for the concept of value pricing.
- In the non-Medicare portion of the plan, the use of formularies, generic substitution, mail-order pharmacies, and drug utilization review was strongly advocated.

## THE RESPONSE TO THE NEW REALITY

While the Clinton Plan never emerged from Congress, anticipation of its effects, combined with other pressures being exerted, resulted in a flurry of activity on the part of or involving the U.S. industry.

The days of annual revenue growth of 15% appear to have become very much a thing of the past. As already noted, cutbacks in the level of price increases were seen. While reaping the improvement in public relations of such action, the industry also "reaped" a substantial slowdown in year-to-year growth. If price increases of necessity contribute less to overall growth, the slack has to be taken up by either increases in unit volume or new product sales. While new product revenue in the U.S. market approached $700 million in 1993, this was barely sufficient to offset the revenue loss in the overall market caused by the ever-increasing penetration of generics with their lower unit prices (1). Unit volume increases were of little substance as a growth factor.

Substantial discounting, or rebating to third-party operations, both public and private, has become more the rule than the exception it had been.

Sweeping layoffs and mandated or "suggested" early retirements are no longer unique occurrences in the pharmaceutical industry. From July of 1993 to January of 1995, 11 major brand manufacturers announced the elimination of a total of 34,000 jobs.

"Restructuring," "rationalization," and "elimination of redundancies" have become primary objectives in the industry, as has "budgetary restraint."

Acquisition activity, after lying fallow for a period, reemerged with a flurry. So, too, did divestiture activity. Roche acquired Syntex. American Home bought American Cyanamid. As of this writing, BASF is negotiating to buy Boots, Glaxo has made an offer to Wellcome, and Hoechst is in discussions with Marion Merrell Dow. Kodak opted to leave the pharmaceutical business, selling the Sterling prescription business to Sanofi, its alliance partner, and the Sterling OTC operation to SmithKline Beecham. SmithKline Beecham subsequently sold to Bayer the Sterling OTC business in North America. The Animal Health Division of SmithKline Beecham was sold to Pfizer.

While the latter buyings and sellings may be labeled as among peers, some members of the brand-name segment of the industry went a bit farther afield and engaged in a flurry of acquisition and other activity related to the generic side of the business. Hoechst acquired Copley. Bayer purchased an interest in Schein. Marion Merrell Dow acquired Rugby. Other brand-name companies entered the generics market via the creation of in-house generic operations: RPR/Arcola, Zeneca/IPR, Schering/Warrick, Upjohn/Greenstone, Syntex/Hamilton, and Merck/West Point Pharma (although the latter two are in the process of being dissolved or phased out). Still others created alliances or licensing relationships with generic companies; examples would be SmithKline Beecham/Rugby and Lilly/Mylan. Such activities were not limited to the U.S. market. As an example, Bristol-Myers Squibb purchased an interest in Azupharma, a German generic company, and there is evidence of brand-name companies looking into the potential of the generic business in Japan.

Perhaps the most surprising step away from historic drug company culture was the acquisition by Merck of Medco, the mail-order pharmacy/pharmacy benefit management operation. Within a year of the Merck/Medco event, other major companies had followed suit in the acquisition of or purchase of significant interest in other pharmacy benefit management companies. Lilly acquired Pharmaceutical Card Services, while SmithKline Beecham did the same with Diversified Pharmaceutical Services.

Another characteristic of the first half of the 1990s was an increased focus on the over-the-counter side of the pharmaceutical business. Transition of prescription-only products to OTC status involved a number of companies and products. Application for such transfer was seen for many drugs in many countries. The $H_2$ antagonists are perhaps the most significant example. While not yet cleared for OTC marketing in the U.S., both Pepcid® and Tagamet® have received such clearance in the U.K. In the U.S., significant drugs approved for OTC status in recent years include naproxen sodium and clemastine fumarate. Also noted during this period were the formation of joint ventures specific to the marketing of OTC drugs; examples are Warner Wellcome and J&J Merck.

While most of the preceding commentary addresses the U.S. market and industry, the conditions described and many of the reactions of the industry are hardly limited to the United States. While the form may vary, the substance of efforts to reduce health care costs and the resultant impact on the industry are noted in virtually every country in the world.

## *INDUSTRY EXPECTATIONS*

A collective view of the actions, reactions, and activities of the pharmaceutical industry in the first half of the 1990s can perhaps be used as a guide to the industry's perception of its structure in the balance of the 1990s and through at least the initial stages of the 21st century. Even the most casual analysis of the occurrences of the past few years suggests the industry expects:

- A redefining of the industry's basic customers
- Continuing but increasingly more stringent efforts at cost containment
- Managed care, managed competition, or increased government intervention as the managers of such cost containment
- An increasing role for generics
- An increasing role for over-the-counter pharmaceuticals
- A need for R&D to provide truly unique and cost-effective drugs
- A substantial slowdown in growth
- A substantial reduction in profitability.

Some thought suggests that the industry's expectations are realistic.

It seems reasonable to expect that the demand for health care in general and medicines in particular will necessarily increase as the population ages. While this expectation may suggest a positive for the industry in terms of increased drug utilization, this increased demand will create an even greater burden on already overstretched health care resources. Measures thus far introduced around the world have been designed to slow down the growth in health care spending without jeopardizing access to or diminishing the quality of health care. But these measures are short term. Further and more drastic measures will be needed in the future.

### Managed Health Care

The industry's expectation of dramatic growth in the importance of managed health care in one form or another appears more than warranted. While the "managers" and the methodologies may differ depending upon country or health care system, the goal of these managers will be to control or cut costs in any way possible. The U.S. market serves as an example for examining the many ramifications of increasing levels of managed health care.

It has been suggested that 90% of the U.S. population will fall under the umbrella of one or another types of managed health care by the end of the decade. The suggestion seems plausible. While Clinton's health reform package, with its orientation to managed care, may be dead, the general concept of health reform–and of managed care as a keystone of such reform–is not. It would be no surprise to find the individual states putting health reform of one variety or another into effect. A number of states (California, Florida, Hawaii, Minnesota, Oregon, Vermont, Washington) have already proposed or put into place programs to expand coverage of their citizens and, at the same time, to reduce health care costs.

IMS estimates that managed health care (public and private) accounted for 73% of pharmaceutical product sales in 1994 and 55% of all new prescriptions in the same year, the latter compared to 37% in 1990 (2). There is little doubt that these shares will move higher over the next few years and may even reach the 90-95% levels by the beginning of the next century.

The impact of managed care on the industry will increase, and it will be multifold.

Attempts by managed care to achieve a reduction in drug costs have taken many routes. As noted earlier, formularies (positive and negative) have been put into place. Mandated generic prescribing by physicians or mandatory generic substitution by pharmacists are other approaches. Use of specific types of prescription dispensers such as mail-order pharmacies is mandated in some cases. The services of pharmacy benefit managers are employed in others. Not uncommon is the concurrent use of more than one of these approaches. As managed care embraces more and more of the market, these attempts at drug cost reduction will proliferate and will strengthen.

The mandating of the prescribing or the dispensing of generics and the expected stricter enforcement of such mandates will have a chilling effect on the brand-name products and companies as well as on growth in the overall market.

It is likely that the bulk of the expected increased demand for drugs will be taken up by generics. In an attempt to quantify this statement, if one were to assume that *all* of the demand for branded products that are *presently* off patent were to be shifted to generics, the result would be a reduction of $11 billion annually in branded product volume but an increase of only $2 billion in generic product revenues. The net loss of $9 billion would reflect a decline of 15% in the size of the U.S. market. It is unlikely that such a shift would take place in a short time period, but the figures do make the point that increased generic penetration severely affects branded product volume and overall market size and growth. The numbers for the future? Between 1994 and the year 2000, patents will expire on products presently in the U.S. market with 1993 sales volume of close to $12 billion (2).

These statistics suggest a rationale for the previously noted move into the generic sector by a number of brand-name companies. There will, undoubtedly, be more such moves, perhaps to the point that the historic distinction between brand and generic companies will cease to exist.

Most formularies will eschew the use of a branded multiple-source product in favor of a generic version, but formularies also address the use of single-source products. It is in formulary systems that even a unique, single-source drug will be required to justify its inclusion on a positive formulary or exclusion from a negative formulary if there are *therapeutically equivalent* products available. While six of the seven ACE inhibitor drugs presently on the U.S. market are single source and are chemically different, it is probably true that most are viewed as therapeutically interchangeable with each other. If one accepts this reasoning, it follows that a primary decision factor as to which of these drugs will win a place on a formulary (assuming a positive formulary) will be price. Thus, while such single-source products may not be subject to *generic equivalent* substitution, they are and will continue to be subjected to a form of *therapeutic* substitution on the basis of price and other factors which will be discussed later. The net result is that these products will be less profitable than might have been expected because there will be a need to compete on price. The breadth of the potential for such therapeutic substitution is illustrated by the fact that of the ten largest dollar-volume categories in drugstores in 1994, all were dominated by therapeutically equivalent drugs (2). Although the point may be argued, these therapeutically equivalent products are, in practical terms, closer to commodity as opposed to unique status, more fungible than not.

As the umbrella of managed care covers more and more of the provision of health care, pharmacy benefit management, already a part of the managed care fabric, will assume an even larger role in the future. Pharmacy benefit managers (PBMs) make the claim that they are capable of effecting considerable savings on pharmaceutical costs via prescription monitoring, pharmacy discounts, and contracted manufacturer rebates. A typical PBM's electronic claims processing system will carry out drug utilization review, check claims, check for drug interactions, determine whether substitution is mandated or permitted, designate copayments, etc. In addition, certain PBMs have instituted their own formulary systems; beneficiaries are given prescribing guidelines to present to their physicians. Another approach is to provide bonuses to pharmacists for dispensing generics, with the bonus generally being a percentage of the savings achieved by use of the generic.

Mail-order pharmacy operations may also be considered a segment of the managed care approach. While initially touted as simply lower cost prescription dispensers, at least some mail-order pharmacy operators have expanded in scope to include benefit management services. Mail-order pharmacy accounted for close to 7% of pharmaceutical dollar volume in 1994 and some 4% of all prescriptions dispensed (2). The rate of growth in the mail-order segment over the past five years has outstripped that of all other prescription dispensing operations. This pattern is expected to continue, as it is estimated that currently fewer than one-third of eligible beneficiaries make use of mail-order pharmacies.

The acquisition of or alliance with pharmacy benefit managers or, as in the case of Medco, mail-order pharmacy/pharmacy benefit managers by pharmaceutical companies was initially viewed with some surprise. While horizontal integration was certainly not new to the industry, vertical integration of the type represented by these acquisitions was.

Ownership of a PBM can open a window of opportunity for a manufacturer to provide more products more frequently to the managed care market. It should also provide the manufacturer with a fund of information and technology with which to monitor patients, to analyze compliance, and to determine outcomes of therapeutic approaches. The possibility of a PBM favoring the manufacturer owner's products, however, appears unlikely. The Federal Trade Commission's investigation of the Lilly/PCS situation resulted in requirements that formularies remain open and that the manufacturer owner be denied access to competitive pricing information. It is likely that such restrictions will be applied to other similar situations such as Merck/Medco and SmithKline Beecham/Diversified. It is expected, however, that alliances with PBMs will be more beneficial than not, in spite of these restrictions.

The concept of disease state management is another phenomenon of the first part of the 1990s. It is also viewed as a part of the managed care picture, although it is certainly not limited to managed care. The concept is essentially predicated upon the limitation of risk to the health care provider or payer by the supplying of a line of therapeutics and other measures designed to treat a disease entity such as diabetes, asthma, or hypertension for a fixed or limited cost. Many manufacturers have announced their intention to provide disease state management; some have gone so far as to create divisions or separate companies to provide such services. The sought-after result here is the use of the guarantor's product or products.

Implicit in a number of the aspects discussed with regard to managed care is the need for the industry to realign its thinking with respect to the question of who its customers are. It appears that the classic industry "customer," the physician, is declining in importance in favor of the HMO, or the PBM, or the state, or the formulary committee, or any number of nonphysicians. It is expected that this will continue to be the case in the future.

Formulary systems, or any system that effectively mandates which drugs or products a physician may or may not prescribe, may have a profound effect on promotional activities in the industry, at least as they are presently known. The simple question that arises here is, If the prescribing physician is not the ultimate decision maker with respect to what he or she prescribes, where is the necessity of promoting the prescribing physician? The reality, of course, is less stark than the question, but it does seem plausible that promotional or educational efforts will have to be directed toward the respective decision makers, whomever and wherever they are. It is certainly the case that the number of these decision makers is considerably less than the number of prescribing physicians in the United States. The latter point would lead to the conclusion that there will be a decline in the costs of promotion incurred by the industry.

In line with an expectation of shifts in the targets for promotion is an expectation that there will be a qualitative change in the conveying of product information. Price will, undoubtedly, assume even greater import as a component of product information, so, too, will the results of outcomes analysis, pharmacoeconomic studies, and the importance of the drug or the drug company's efforts in the disease management context. The costs involved in the performance of such analyses or studies, of course, may negate the savings hypothesized by the need to promote to fewer decision makers.

### *The Over-the-Counter Market*

The increased focus on the over-the-counter side of the pharmaceutical business was commented on earlier. While it has historically been the case that movement of a product from prescription-only status to OTC status results in increased sales volume, there are other rationales for moving to the over-the-counter, or nonprescription, side. Major among these are cost-containment implications and the generic situation.

The cost-containment factor is related to the concept of cost shifting. One method health care providers and payers use to contain costs is to move the patient from a covered prescription drug to an uncovered nonprescription medication. The cost thus shifts from the payer to the patient. There are two competing scenarios potentially at work here. One involves the patient who responds to the OTC concept because it means no physician visit, for which he or she might pay in full or in part, and the probable lesser financial outlay for an OTC as opposed to a prescription drug if prescriptions are paid for in full or in part by the patient. The other scenario consists of the patient whose physician visits and prescription costs are fully covered and who might balk at having to pay for an uncovered OTC product. The issue, of course, could be forced by the payers.

The generic factor enters into the OTC situation in the sense of a form of exclusivity protection. If, in the United States, a manufacturer succeeds in obtaining approval for an OTC version of a prescription drug, that manufacturer is assured of a three-year exclusivity period for the OTC version. Therefore, if a manufacturer can successfully switch prescription business for the drug to OTC business, generic competition can be forestalled for the three-year period.

Both rationales suggest further emphasis on the OTC market by the industry. However, it is questionable whether the OTC market will grow to the size some predict as a result of prescription-to-OTC transitions. While antiulcerants such as Tagamet, Pepcid, and Zantac® do represent enormous potential for the OTC market, none of the other billion-dollar categories in the U.S. market–except for NSAIDs–would appear likely to offer Rx-to-OTC potential. It is unlikely, for example, that an OTC ace inhibitor is in anyone's future.

It is likely that the high level of investment needed to compete in the OTC sector will cause consolidation in this sector of the business. Small companies without niche products likely will not be able to compete. Prescription-driven companies lacking critical mass in OTCs will seek strategic alliances or partnerships with consumer product oriented competitors, à la Wellcome with Warner-Lambert.

### Research and Development

Pressures on research and development, in the context of slimmer pipelines or the inability to achieve critical mass in terms of investment capability, are certainly one factor in the relatively recent wave of merger and acquisition activity. New products have historically been the lifeblood of the pharmaceutical industry. They will continue to be so. However, lower profitability in the wake of cost containment measures is likely to cause a decline in any growth in R&D spending. It also seems apparent that R&D will become increasingly expensive as a result of the increased pressure to produce significant, cost-justifiable new entities and new technologies, not merely derivatives or spin-offs of already available therapy.

It is expected that there will be increased pressure not only to produce unique and significant entities but also to move these entities through research much more quickly. Beyond the more obvious reasons, there is the possibility that the imposition of requirements for outcomes analysis will lengthen the period before a new product will be accepted for use on a formulary or by a payer or provider.

There is an obvious circularity in the R&D situation. R&D will need to produce more significant products more quickly; thus, it will become more difficult and more expensive. At the same time, a decline is expected in the profitability of the industry, resulting in less money to invest in R&D.

Methods of dealing with the R&D problem will probably include an increase in the alignments of pharmaceutical manufacturers with the biotechnology sector. Many such alliances presently exist. Of close to 400 pharmaceutical R&D alliances presently identifiable, 200 are with biotechnology firms. More will be seen in the future.

More decentralizing of R&D activities will likely be seen, along with more reliance on the "outsourcing" of some of these activities to independent contract research organizations, the latter more in the realm of "development" than "research." Another possibility is more merger or acquisition activity involving major firms.

Somewhat tangential to the R&D question is the question of licensing. A large number of very successful products presently in the U.S. market have not been researched or developed by the companies marketing them. These products, instead, have been licensed for sale in the U.S. from their originators, in many cases, Japanese companies. A significant number of U.S. companies, large and small, have not engaged in full-scale R&D activity but have achieved success by licensing products for the U.S. market.

Licensing as an avenue to success may not constitute a particularly viable option in the future. If, as expected, new therapies become harder to develop, the originating company may be less likely to license such therapies. This would be the case especially if non-U.S. companies, from which many of the licenses are obtained, choose to extend their business into other countries.

## THE INDUSTRY OF THE FUTURE

Where does this review of the present and of industry's expectations of the future lead us with respect to characterizing the structure of the industry into the next century?

In general terms, for the industry and its participants to be successful in the future, the industry will have to understand that it cannot view itself or the therapies it provides as a distinct part of the health care picture. The successful company of the future will be the company that undertakes to participate in the provision of cost-effective health care to the utmost degree possible.

It is expected that the next 10 to 15 years will see the industry's macro responses to the pressures being exerted upon it as including:

- Strategically adjacent collaboration
- Integration with payers and providers
- Strategic investment in research and development companies
- Integration of production and supply
- Maximization of process efficiencies
- Product life cycle management.

It seems as well that companies will have to decide what role they will play in the market of the future or, in other words, the character of their mission. Major options for choice would likely include:

- A prescription product centered, integrated health care supplier
- An integrated provider of cost-effective solutions to health care management/cost containment
- A research and development based source of unique therapeutics.

The responses and the possible choices implicitly argue for streamlining and consolidation, with the likely result that the industry will be a much smaller industry in terms of the number of firms participating. While the pharmaceutical industry of the future may not quite resemble the automobile industry in the United States, with its 3 major companies, the next century may see as few as 10 to 15 major companies constituting the pharmaceutical industry. Like the auto industry, there may be a number of divisions within each company, but the corporate entities will be much reduced in number.

These corporate entities will likely encompass much more than the typical drug company of the past. There may be a branded product operation, a generic operation, a distribution component, an OTC segment, a disease management division, etc., that are not necessarily separate entities, but, instead, integrated so as to provide the services, cost efficiencies, and value-added component that will be required by the ultimate health care payers.

Those companies that do possess a generic operation will attempt to capitalize on one of the major strengths of the previously independent generic companies–excellent distribution scope–and may move into lines of business that can take advantage of such distribution networks.

The industry of the future will be characterized by a much greater number of strategic alliances than is the case today. To the degree that the corporate entity does not or cannot afford to embrace necessary activities or functions, it will look to others, either in the industry or outside, to provide these efforts. These alliances or joint ventures will take many forms. A company may ally with another drug company or a biotechnology company for research purposes. It might contract with an outside organization for development work. It may launch a joint venture with a consumer-oriented company. The need for information for outcomes research, or patient monitoring, or epidemiologic studies might involve alliances with others who possess such information. There will be an increase in the number of the already familiar alliances for marketing and promotion, as well. Independent contract organizations will become much more significant as partners to the industry as "outsourcing" of many activities will be viewed by the industry as desirable or necessary.

The next 10 to 15 years will see a marked departure from historical methods and approaches to the promotion or advertising of products, both quantitative and qualitative. Sales force sizes will decline, and the role of the professional representative will change. The professional representative of the next century will be schooled not only in the efficacy of the products he or she is discussing but also in their cost efficiency. His or her audience will no longer consist exclusively of the prescriber but will consist much more of the managed care decision makers, whoever and wherever these might be.

Product claims of efficacy or superiority per se will no longer be accepted on the largely *ipse dixit* basis that has been the case historically. It will have to be proven that such is the case, and such proof will have to originate in the larger arenas of positive outcomes, cost-effectiveness, and role in disease management, as well as in what the product is pharmacologically capable of doing.

The industry has long been characterized as one that had very little contact with its ultimate consumer–the patient. This will change. Seeds of this change are already apparent, one example being the area of prostatic hypertrophy. Direct-to-consumer, or patient, advertising and education can result in additional sales for a drug. Just as important, it can promote consumer awareness of a potential health problem and thus represent a benefit in overall health care terms.

The industry is coming to understand that there is a consumer-driven aspect, even to the prescription product side of the business, and the future will see more efforts to "get closer" to the consumer, whether an individual patient, an employer, an HMO, etc.

It is expected that the 21st century industry will be much more heavily involved in those areas of the world presently identified under the banner of "emerging markets"–Eastern Europe, Southeast Asia, etc. While not necessarily free of risk in commercial and economic terms, these markets will offer much needed growth potential.

There are, no doubt, many other changes that will be noted in the industry of the next century compared to the industry of today. The ones suggested above are those that come most readily to mind.

A few final comments.

While much of the preceding analysis/prediction focuses on the U.S. market in the sense of example, it is to be reiterated that, although *form* may differ, the substance of changes now occurring and changes in the future will apply to the entirety of the marketplace, not just the United States.

The scenarios depicted may be altered to some degree by discoveries of better treatments or curative agents for the more difficult diseases, such as AIDS and cancer. Predictions of much-slowed growth rates, for example, would be altered by such discoveries.

Lastly, it is to be hoped, if not predicted, that the industry of the future will achieve more success in conveying to its customers, whomever they may be, that without the pharmaceutical industry and its discoveries, the cost in lives, in quality of lives, and in financial terms would be absolutely unfathomable.

## REFERENCES

1. The U.S. year in review. IMS International, 1993.
2. The U.S. year in review. IMS International, 1994.

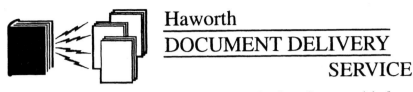

# Haworth
# DOCUMENT DELIVERY
## SERVICE

This valuable service provides a single-article order form for any article from a Haworth journal.

- *Time Saving:* No running around from library to library to find a specific article.
- *Cost Effective:* All costs are kept down to a minimum.
- *Fast Delivery:* Choose from several options, including same-day FAX.
- *No Copyright Hassles:* You will be supplied by the original publisher.
- *Easy Payment:* Choose from several easy payment methods.

---

*Open Accounts Welcome for ...*
- Library Interlibrary Loan Departments
- Library Network/Consortia Wishing to Provide Single-Article Services
- Indexing/Abstracting Services with Single Article Provision Services
- Document Provision Brokers and Freelance Information Service Providers

---

### MAIL or *FAX* THIS ENTIRE ORDER FORM TO:

Haworth Document Delivery Service
The Haworth Press, Inc.
10 Alice Street
Binghamton, NY 13904-1580

or FAX: 1-800-895-0582
or CALL: 1-800-342-9678
9am-5pm EST

---

PLEASE SEND ME PHOTOCOPIES OF THE FOLLOWING SINGLE ARTICLES:

1) Journal Title: _____
   Vol/Issue/Year: _____ Starting & Ending Pages: _____
   Article Title: _____
   _____

2) Journal Title: _____
   Vol/Issue/Year: _____ Starting & Ending Pages: _____
   Article Title: _____
   _____

3) Journal Title: _____
   Vol/Issue/Year: _____ Starting & Ending Pages: _____
   Article Title: _____
   _____

4) Journal Title: _____
   Vol/Issue/Year: _____ Starting & Ending Pages: _____
   Article Title: _____
   _____

**(See other side for Costs and Payment Information)**

**COSTS:** Please figure your cost to order quality copies of an article.

1. Set-up charge per article: $8.00

($8.00 × number of separate articles) _____

2. Photocopying charge for each article:

1-10 pages: $1.00 _____

11-19 pages: $3.00 _____

20-29 pages: $5.00 _____

30+ pages: $2.00/10 pages _____

3. Flexicover (optional): $2.00/article _____

4. Postage & Handling: US: $1.00 for the first article/

$.50 each additional article _____

Federal Express: $25.00 _____

Outside US: $2.00 for first article/

$.50 each additional article_____

5. Same-day FAX service: $.35 per page _____

**GRAND TOTAL:** _____

---

**METHOD OF PAYMENT:** (please check one)

❑ Check enclosed ❑ Please ship and bill. PO # _____

(sorry we can ship and bill to bookstores only! All others must pre-pay)

❑ Charge to my credit card: ❑ Visa; ❑ MasterCard; ❑ Discover;
❑ American Express;

Account Number:_____ Expiration date:_____

Signature: X_____

Name: _____ Institution: _____

Address: _____

_____

City: _____ State:_____ Zip:_____

Phone Number: _____ FAX Number: _____

---

## MAIL or *FAX* THIS ENTIRE ORDER FORM TO:

| Haworth Document Delivery Service | **or FAX:** 1-800-895-0582 |
| The Haworth Press, Inc. | **or CALL:** 1-800-342-9678 |
| 10 Alice Street | 9am-5pm EST) |
| Binghamton, NY 13904-1580 | |